An Holistic Guide to Reflexology

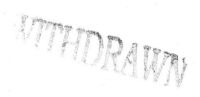

Hairdressing And Beauty Industry Authority Series – related titles

An Holistic Guide to Reflexology

Tina Parsons

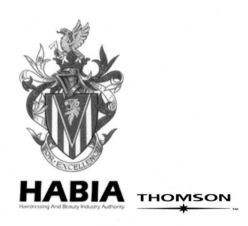

HABIA
Hairdressing And Beauty Industry Authority

THOMSON ™

Australia • Canada • Mexico • Singapore • Spain • United Kingdom • United States

THOMSON

An Holistic Guide to Reflexology

Copyright © Tina Parsons 2003

The Thomson logo is a trademark used herein under licence.

For more information, contact Thomson Learning, High Holborn House, 50–51 Bedford Row, London, WC1R 4LR or visit us on the World Wide Web at: http://www.thomsonlearning.co.uk

British Library Cataloguing in Publication Data
A catalogue record for this book is available from the British Library

ISBN 1-86152-907-4

Typeset by 𝒯 Tek-Art, Croydon, Surrey

Printed and bound in Croatia by Zrinski

Contents

Foreword

When it comes to relaxing, having a reflexology session would always be on the top of my list. I've found reflexology to be a fascinating subject. As a client at the receiving end of reflexology, I've always felt rewarded and revitalised after each session. So much so, that I was keen for the HABIA/Thomson Learning partnership to create the best-ever guide on the subject. I'm delighted to say that Tina Parsons has created a masterpiece beyond my expectations.

I first met Tina when HABIA started work on the new Beauty Therapy Standards in 1998. Tina was one of the industry experts who immediately came to mind when we started to devise the national structure for NVQs. Tina impressed me straight away with her quiet yet determined manner and her tremendous passion and knowledge of the industry.

As a National Training Award winner in 1999 and 2000, and a multiple winner of numerous beauty awards, I couldn't think of anyone else who was better qualified to write this excellent holistic guide to reflexology.

Alan Goldsbro
Chief Executive Officer
Hairdressing And Beauty Industry Authority

Introduction

Learning does not take place in isolation, nor does it happen without any prior knowledge. Learning occurs when intuition combines with tuition and the inspiration for this book lies with all the students, staff and clients who have ever asked me for more – more reasons why, more explanations where and more descriptions how? May you never cease to ask questions!

This book has therefore been written in a quest to address the many and varied questions that accompany a course of reflexology. It provides a starting point for beginners with the traditional method of foot reflexology. It contains suitable reference for qualified practitioners seeking to refresh their knowledge and encourages the development of advanced reflexology techniques with methods for hand and ear reflexology. In addition, it will make interesting reading for clients, helping to promote understanding and awareness.

The book has been divided into four parts:

1. The facts
2. The skills
3. The consultation
4. The treatment

Each part has been subdivided into chapters for ease of study and to provide further detailed information. Within the text, words in bold type alert the reader to important points or terms which are then explained. They are included in the glossary where appropriate.

In addition, there is the inclusion of easy to follow guides in the form of **system sorter**, **common conditions**, **order of work**, **treatment tracker**, **holistic harmony**, **case study** and **colour plates**.

- **System sorter** is a quick and easy guide to the way in which the systems of the body depend on one another for their well-being. The links between the individual systems are highlighted, encouraging a more holistic viewpoint.

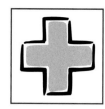

- **Common conditions** provides information on a variety of conditions common to each system of the body together with the suggested direct and indirect reflexes.
- **Order of work** provides a step-by-step guide to treatment of the feet, hands and ears together with detailed diagrams of the reflexes for each body system.
- **Treatment tracker** includes a quick and easy guide to the way in which reflexology can be adapted to incorporate the treatment of the **zones, meridians** and **chakras** on the **feet, hands** and **ears** with the use of **visualisation, affirmation, colour** and **sound**.

- **Holistic harmony** includes information about the needs of the body systems and is subdivided into eight different categories including **air, water, nutrition, rest, activity, ageing, awareness** and **special care**. This section provides information that forms the basis for aftercare advice given at the end of the treatment.
- **Case Study** offers information on a variety of common objectives, expectations and outcomes of reflexology treatments.
- **Colour plates** map out the reflexes on each foot, hand and ear for easy reference.

Fascinating facts are included throughout the text, highlighting special areas of interest.

Angel advice aims to provide a source of inspiration with a thought or a deed that continues the concept of effective teaching and learning by building awareness, seeking development and initiating changes.

At the end of each chapter there is an opportunity to check your learning with **tasks** and **knowledge reviews**.

- **Tasks** are included with each chapter to enhance your theoretical and practical skills through research and development.

- **Knowledge review** provides the opportunity to test your knowledge with a set of short answer questions. The questions are designed to ensure that you have gained the appropriate level of understanding of the theory that underpins reflexology.

Activities are included throughout the text, encouraging practical participation and experiential learning.

Tip and **remember** boxes help you to recall and understand the main points concerned with system and treatment linking.

Website

In addition to the information provided by the book, there is also access to an interactive website for students and lecturer's to use. The website will provide a back-up to learning by supplying the answers to the **Knowledge review** questions as well as multiple choice questions for each chapter. It has been designed to provide as much access to varied learning as possible in an attempt to meet the growing needs of individual learners. Lecturer support will also be provided in the form of interactive input facilitating the use of techniques for teaching, assessing and checking the learning process.

Acknowledgements

Once again I have appreciated the opportunity that Thomson have given me to write this book, and would like to dedicate it to my daughter Alexa as she takes her first steps into the art and science that is reflexology.

Tina Parsons
2002

Part 1
The basics

Learning objectives

After reading this part you should be able to:

- Recognise the areas of the body where reflexology can be used.

- Identify the different theories that contribute to the art and science of reflexology.

- Understand the links between the different theories and reflexology.

- Be aware of the ancient and modern historical origins of reflexology.

- Begin to appreciate the links between reflexology and healing.

Reflexology is at the same time both a simple and a complex form of holistic therapy.

The literal translations of these terms can help in our understanding of the treatment:

- Reflex – reflected;
- Ology – the study of;
- Holistic – the whole person;
- Therapy – healing.

Reflexology therefore incorporates the study of a part of the body that is able to reflect all other parts in order to bring about healing of the whole of a human being.

There are many parts of the body that are able to provide a reflection of the human being including cells and organs, but areas such as the feet, hands and ears are excellent examples of external body parts that are more easily accessible for treatment. Because of this mirror imagery any healing that takes place therefore has the potential to incorporate all aspects of the whole person including body, mind and spirit.

Reflexology

 Angel advice

Think about how the art of touch makes you feel. This will help you to appreciate where you are as a person in terms of the use of touch. If the thought of touching other people fills you with feelings of embarrassment, discomfort or even distaste then you have a longer journey to follow than those of you who feel comfortable with the thought of touch.

 Angel advice

A reflexology practitioner should ensure that they are both competent and confident in their knowledge and skill prior to working on members of the public.

In its simplest form reflexology is an intuitive skill and one to which everyone has access from the moment they are born. We can all apply pressure techniques to our own bodies including our feet, hands and ears and in doing so improve our general sense of well-being. We are able to do this as required without even thinking about it, and without having any real knowledge of what we are doing except that it feels good! On this basic level we are also well equipped to practise such skills on our loved ones to bring about a sense of healing.

 Activity

The art of touch is the science of love. Take time to think about the reactions you get when you intuitively touch yourself or another person. Think how powerful the reactions can be in terms of stimulating, soothing, caring and calming – all of which are vital forms of healing.

In its most complex form reflexology works on many different levels, evolving from a long history incorporating a variety of theories and attitudes, methods and practices in order to offer a professional service to achieve specific healing objectives. Many of these are acquired skills that involve specific training for the practitioner to become competent. Some require a whole new mindset and therefore substantial experiential learning before the practitioner is confident to apply the skills on other people.

The history of reflexology

Reflexology has both Western and Eastern origins, sharing its development with a number of different and ancient cultures. No one culture or period in history can claim to be the founder of reflexology, yet all civilisations throughout time have contributed to the art and science that is the reflexology of today. Throughout history we can find many parallels and times when different cultures, far removed from one another, were involved in the development of the same theories and practices, albeit in different ways.

Ancient history

We can track the origins of reflexology from ancient Egypt, migrating over the centuries to Greece, Arabia and on to Europe through the Roman Empire. At the same time we can also find historical evidence of reflexology in ancient India. The religious studies of Hinduism and Buddhism demonstrate the healing beliefs of the time, which can be tracked through to China and Japan with the migration of Buddhist monks. There is also strong Native American evidence to back up their claims for ownership of reflexology. To substantiate these claims historians have found primary sources of evidence from:

- Paintings in Egyptian tombs from as far back as 2500 BC depicting the giving and receiving of treatments to various parts of the body including the hands, feet and ears.

- Stone carvings found in India, China and Japan showing identical features relating to healing through specific body parts e.g. the feet.

- The use of pressure massage to the feet, hands and ears as a form of healing has been passed from generation to generation of Buddhist monks in India, China and Japan as well as through the tribes of Native Americans.

- Explorers and travellers of these times were able to relay by word of mouth the practices seen at first hand in foreign

Tip

Microcosm = miniature
                representation
                of a larger
                system.
Macrocosm = large system.

parts. This led to a gradual and cumulative linking and merging of influences throughout the world.

In addition, the many forms of secondary sources include:

● Historical and medical books as well as religious writings tracking the development of healing theories through the cultures and the centuries.

Although there is very little primary evidence left in existence and gaps and inconsistencies emerge from the secondary evidence, the results are nonetheless conclusive in their own right.

The strong evidence gleaned from ancient history leads us to believe that a common theory developed amongst people all over the world. There was shared belief that there existed in each person a miniature representation of the whole body – in some theories, the whole universe. The feet, hands and ears feature highly throughout these ancient times as examples of microcosms reflecting the macrocosm that is the human body, with reflexology emerging as an ancient form of healing.

 Fascinating Fact

Acupuncture means 'needle piercing'. It incorporates the use of very fine needles inserted into the skin to stimulate specific points called acupoints to aid healing and is a popular treatment today.

 Fascinating Fact

Iridology is the study of how the iris of the eye relates to all parts of the body. The eye is therefore an example of a microcosm reflecting the macrocosm that is the whole person.

The Eastern cultures went on to discover their own systems of healing, far removed from some of those that developed in the West:

● The Chinese discovered a method of medicine that centred on the flow of energy along meridians or pathways within the body. They referred to this energy as **'chi'**. Access to the meridians was developed through acupuncture.

● The Japanese developed a method of holistic therapy they called shiatsu which incorporated the application of manual pressure to points along the meridians called 'tsubo'. They used the term **'ki'** to describe energy.

● Ayurvedic medicine developed in India where energy was identified as **prana**. Chakras or energy centres formed the special points where energy lines or **nadis** crossed and could be activated through touch.

 Fascinating Fact

Shiatsu means 'finger pressure' and can be described as acupuncture without needles. It is a technique much in use today in massage treatments worldwide.

 Fascinating Fact

Ayurveda means 'the science of life' and incorporates an holistic approach to living to which many people aspire.

Modern history

What followed was a period of continued cultural development, with the emergence of a distinct divide between Eastern and Western cultures.

The well-defined healing systems of Eastern cultures continued to develop whilst in Europe the beginning of modern history saw the development of science and the separation of the study of the body and the mind. This resulted in a less holistic approach to healing than that which had emerged from ancient times and rapid medical advancement began to take place. The physical, quantifiable field of study proved to be more popular at the time, although there is some evidence of advancements in reflexology in the Western world. This was associated with the study of the nervous system in the latter part of the nineteenth and early part of the twentieth century. The discovery of reflex actions in relation to the central nervous system proved that there was a neurological link between the external organ of the skin and the internal organs of the body. The development of these theories can be traced throughout Europe. Scientists from Britain, Germany and Russia developed quantifiable evidence to support the theory that parts of the body could be stimulated indirectly through the application of pressure to other areas of the body, thus providing an unquestionable link within the body as a whole.

- In Britain Sir Henry Head developed 'Head's zones', charting areas of the skin that affected internal areas of the body through the nervous system.
- Another Britain, Sir Charles Sherrington, explored the responses made by the nervous system to external stimuli.
- Edgar Adrian shared the Nobel Prize with Sherrington for their work on the nervous system. Adrian went on to demonstrate that the intensity of nerve impulse depended on the size of the nerve and not the strength of the stimulus.
- In Germany Dr Alfons Cornelius discovered that not only did localised areas of sensitivity respond to pressure but that the application of pressure also had an effect in other areas of the body, bringing about changes.
- Russian doctors, Ivan Sechenov and Nobel Prize winner Ivan Pavlov, both studied reflex actions and the correlation between an external stimulus and an internal response.

This research precipitated the development of dermatomes or segmented regions of the body each of which are supplied with a spinal or cranial nerve, thus linking the body with the brain and vice versa.

Reflexology was formally developed into a science in the modern world in the early part of the twentieth century. This development can be tracked through the works of a number of influential American medical practitioners:

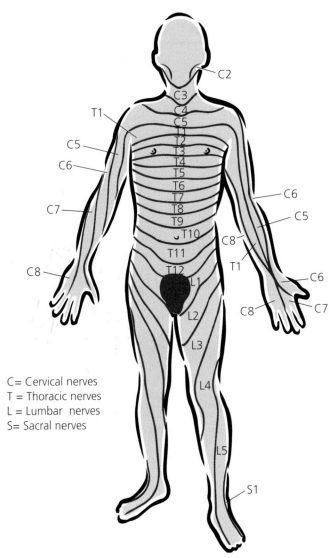

C2
C3
C4
C5
T1
T2
T3
T4
T5
T6
T7
T8
T9
T10
T11
T12
T1
C5
C6
C7
C8
C6
C5
C8
T1
C6
C8
C7
L1
L2
L3
L4
L5
S1

C= Cervical nerves
T = Thoracic nerves
L = Lumbar nerves
S= Sacral nerves

Dermatomes

- Dr William Fitzgerald is thought to have been influenced by a number of medical publications from central Europe whilst working in Vienna in the early 1900s specialising in the treatment of the ear, nose and throat. Whether he also had knowledge of the origins and parallels of reflexology through ancient history and Eastern cultures is unclear. On his return to America, Dr Fitzgerald experimented with the application of pressure to various points in the nose, mouth and throat for pain relief. He went on to discover that he could 'map out' corresponding areas of the body into ten longitudinal **zones**. He found that by applying pressure on various parts of the body, e.g. the hands and the feet, he could induce the relief of pain in a corresponding part within each zone. He used non-electrical applicators to vary the pressure including metal combs, probes, pegs and rubber bands. As a result he was able to formally introduce zone therapy as a science. In itself this was not a new concept, but it heralded the start of the links between Eastern and Western beliefs.

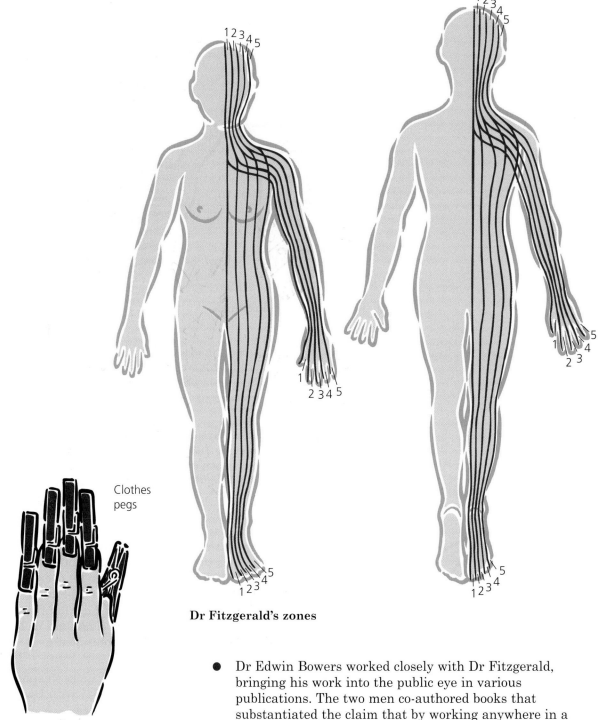

Dr Fitzgerald's zones

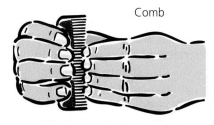

Clothes pegs

Comb

Non-electrical applicators

- Dr Edwin Bowers worked closely with Dr Fitzgerald, bringing his work into the public eye in various publications. The two men co-authored books that substantiated the claim that by working anywhere in a zone, everything else in the same zone was affected. Their claims were met with fierce opposition from fellow medical practitioners, despite the fact that the same concepts were being used in other parts of the world.

- Dr Joseph Shelby Riley was one of the few at the time who did believe in zone therapy, which he had learned from Dr Fitzgerald. Dr Riley went on to work out the finer points, making the first detailed maps of the reflexes on the feet and adding eight horizontal zones to Dr Fitzgerald's ten

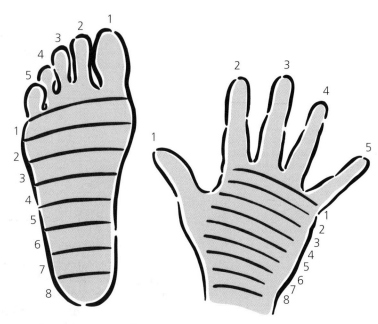

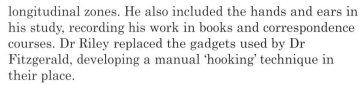

Dr Riley's zones and reflexes

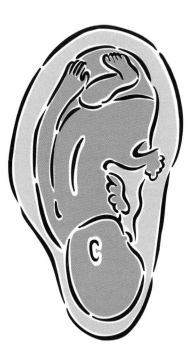

The inverted foetus

longitudinal zones. He also included the hands and ears in his study, recording his work in books and correspondence courses. Dr Riley replaced the gadgets used by Dr Fitzgerald, developing a manual 'hooking' technique in their place.

● Eunice Ingham, a physiotherapist who worked closely with Dr Riley in the early 1930s, became a pioneer of the treatment. She made a distinct separation between work on reflex points and zone therapy, developing what she called compression therapy before renaming it reflexology. Working on hundreds of Dr Riley's patients, she found that an alternating pressure had the effect of stimulating healing and shared this concept with other therapists specialising in areas such as massage, physiotherapy, chiropody, osteopathy etc. Eunice lectured for over thirty years, gaining considerable expertise and experience which she retold in her books, *Stories the Feet Can Tell* first published in 1938 and *Stories the Feet Have Told* in 1951. Her work formed a major part of the treatment as we know it today.

● Dwight Byers and Eusebia Messenger, Eunice's nephew and niece, joined her lecture circuit in 1947 with Dwight continuing her work after her death in 1974.

● Doreen Bayly was trained by Eunice Ingham and was responsible for bringing reflexology to Great Britain in 1966.

● At the same time as Eunice Ingham was developing foot reflexology, scientific investigations were taking place in France into reflexology of the ear. In the late 1950s, Dr Paul Nogier identified corresponding points between the ear and various parts of the body based on the concept of the inverted foetus. He produced the first Western 'map' of the ear.

- Dr Nogier's work was translated into Chinese in 1958 and studies carried out by Nanking Army Ear Acupuncture Research Team were able to verify the accuracy of his map with that of Chinese acupuncture.
- The World Health Organisation (WHO) standardised the use of reflexology and acupuncture to the ear. As a result, ear reflexology, auricular therapy or auriculotherapy (as it is also known) have since evolved from a combination of both Eastern and Western theories.

Today

Angel advice

It is useful to remember that reflexology should be regarded as complementary to the work of the medical profession.

The 'having it all' syndrome associated with recent years has led to increasing stress levels for everyone. As men have experienced changing roles resulting from having to compete with their competent female counterparts they have seen their stress levels rise. Women have also experienced the effects of excessive stress as they attempt to be all things for all people in their quest to become the perfect wife/partner, mother, homemaker and career woman. Children growing up in 'this all or nothing' environment have also experienced raised stress levels, as have the elderly. Children are expected to become high achievers from an increasingly early age and the pressures on the elderly to age well are all factors that have the potential to create unsafe levels of stress. As a result many people have suffered from stress-related illnesses in the form of physical, psychological and spiritual imbalance. The tradition of the medical profession treating the part and not the whole, or the symptom and not the cause has led to a number of people seeking complementary medicine/therapy as a supplement and/or in some cases an alternative. As a result of treating a part that reflects the whole of the body, physical, emotional and spiritual balance has become an achievable aim and reflexology has been able to take its place amongst the more accepted holistic treatments, emerging as a successful and increasingly popular way of combating the stresses of every day life.

Knowledge review

1   What is the literal meaning of reflexology?

2   What do the feet, hands and ears represent in reflexology?

3   Give three areas of the ancient world that can claim to have a reflexology tradition.

4   Name the terms used to describe energy as part of traditional Chinese medicine, Japanese shiatsu and Indian Ayurvedic medicine.

5   What are dermatomes?

6   Who discovered the longitudinal zones as part of zone therapy?

7   What did Dr Riley add to the longitudinal zones?

8   Who developed reflexology from zone therapy?

9   Who developed the inverted foetus theory of ear reflexology?

10   Why is reflexology classified as being a complementary treatment?

2

Theories and attitudes

Theories

The history surrounding the development of reflexology has produced different theories emerging from the different cultures including the theories relating to **zones**, **reflexes**, **meridians** and **chakras**.

Zones and zone therapy

The theory of zones and zone therapy works on the basis of ten main longitudinal zones running through the body. Studies by Dr Fitzgerald and his contemporaries found that applying pressure within the zones reduced or even cut off pain through nerve reflexes before it reaches the brain. This theory is substantiated by scientific research undertaken by Sir Henry Head and Sir Charles Sherrington. Head was able to prove that a connection existed between the skin and the organs of the body via the nervous

 Fascinating Fact

Zone theory can be used in the simplest of circumstances e.g. having recently had to have a potentially painful injection to numb my thumb prior to having the skin stitched I asked my husband to press down firmly on my big toe instead of holding my other hand as he would be inclined to do in such a situation. As a result I experienced less pain, my husband felt useful and the nurse administering the injection was able to complete the task with greater ease! In theory I could have gone ahead and had the skin stitched without the injection, but I would have had an interesting task convincing the nurse of a busy A&E dept!

system; Sherrington discovered that the whole nervous system is able to adjust to stimuli and coordinate the activities within the whole body as a result e.g. changes in body temperature, blood pressure etc.

The theory of reflexes and reflexology

This maps out the organs and systems of the body within the zones, which in turn are also represented on areas such as the feet, hands and ears. Dr Riley's studies supported this theory and Eunice Ingham was instrumental in developing it further, discovering that the application of alternating pressure to specific reflex points on the feet had a stimulating effect on the corresponding body part. This could be achieved through the reflex action associated with the nervous system as well as the stimulation of the circulation in the skin via capillaries that extend internally into the body via larger vessels linking with the heart, lungs and all other organs and systems.

Traditional Chinese medicine and Japanese Shiatsu

These share the theory of fourteen main pairs of meridians or pathways running through the body. The Chinese and Japanese believe that the meridians form a single system that links the body and its parts with the universe through the free flow of energy. Illness occurs when the energy cannot flow freely, becoming blocked and in turn affecting all corresponding body parts of the associated meridians.

Ayurvedic medicine

The Ayurvedic medicine of India works on the theory of seven main chakras or energy centres. It goes beyond the physical, stating that there is more to a human being than just the body and that the chakras provide the link. Energy is able to enter and exit the body via these chakras with the flow of energy affecting the well-being of the person.

Fascinating Fact

Because of the arrangement of nerves in the central nervous system the left brain controls the right side of the body and the right brain controls the left side of the body.

Whilst we can see that there are many similarities between the different theories, there are also apparent discrepancies. Although there are parallels between the zones and meridians and reflexes and chakras, zones and reflexes tend to be associated with the nervous system and meridians and chakras with the energy system. In the past this has caused a split between the development of Western and Eastern methods of healing and created the divide between the science of the West and the art of the East.

However, a bond has begun to form between the theories resulting from open-minded individuals seeking a more balanced answer to healing. The answer lies in the brain, the most complex organ of the body. The brain forms part of the central nervous system. The forebrain or cerebrum is divided into the left and right cerebral hemispheres, also known as the **left brain** and **right brain**.

Left brain

The left brain is responsible for analytical functions and logical thinking. It is associated with the accumulation of knowledge and controls the *right* side of the body.

Right brain

The right brain is responsible for systemic functions and creative thinking. It is associated with intuition and controls the *left* side of the body.

The left and right brain are linked by the corpus callosum allowing the two regions to communicate and coordinate. The two sides of the brain complement each other harmoniously and in order to lead a well-balanced life human beings need to make use of both sides of the brain. Research has found that every person has a predisposition towards greater activity in one side of the brain than the other i.e. they have a dominant and a non-dominant side.

Predominantly left brain people are logical thinkers and tend to be extroverted in personality. They are gifted at languages and exact sciences. They have a good memory for verbal images. Predominantly right brain people, on the other hand, are more perceptive and have a tendency towards a more introverted

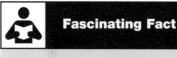
Fascinating Fact

The Western tradition of wanting to test every theory makes it a more left-brain culture, whilst the intuitive action of the Eastern traditions make them more right-brain cultures.

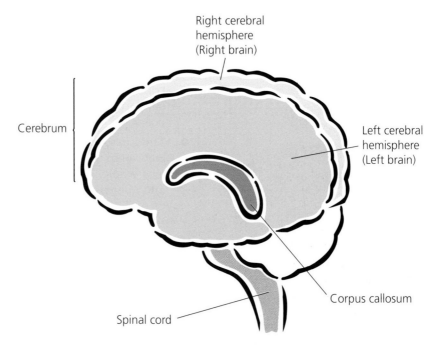

The brain

personality type. Their gifts lie with the arts such as music, dance, painting etc. and they have a natural aptitude for sound.

In the 1960s further research led to the development of the left and right brain type theory. There emerged a theory known as Lafontaine's Principle which stated that:

- People with left brain dominance can be classified as **visual types**. They have acute central vision, i.e. good vision both internally and externally, and are drawn instinctively towards colours.
- People with right brain dominance are **auditory types**. They have a selective ear and analyse and reproduce sound with precision and ease.

Visual type

These people respond instinctively to what they see and the skills associated with visual expertise are dominant.

Auditory type

These people respond instinctively to what they hear and the skills associated with creative expertise are dominant.

Our types are determined by the instinctive responses that emerge as a result of activity in the dominant side of our brains. However, training, will power and reasoning can produce less spontaneous responses and provide us with the means to promote more balanced activity in the brain.

This theory is supported by the Western and Eastern theories of energy incorporating:

- The Western science of energy associated with electrical impulses within the nervous system and the chemical transportation within the circulatory system. This theory supports our left brain activity and appeals to our visual needs.
- The Eastern art of energy associated with the physical, emotional and spiritual interconnection with the universe as a whole. This theory supports our right brain activity and appeals to our auditory needs.

Energy

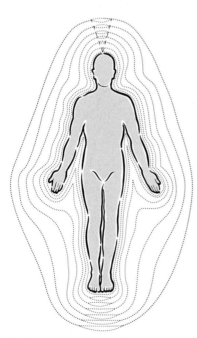

The human energy field – auras

Energy may be described as 'power which may be translated into motion'. The universal energy field (UEF) is associated with the world around us and the human energy field (HEF) with the energy surrounding living things. This is also known as the **aura** and is believed to radiate outwards up to one metre from the body.

Fascinating Fact

Kirlian photography is a method of photographing the HEF to determine the quality of the energy surrounding a person by producing a black and white image. Further scientific advancements have made it possible to produce colour images of the aura. Electrostatic energy, e.g. sound and vibrations in the body, are translated into colour.

Energy is all around us and within us. It is not always visible yet it affects every one of our cells and every aspect of our lives. Light and sound are forms of energy and thus have a powerful influence on our well-being.

Activity

Visualise the energy that has to be produced both internally and externally to create a movement. Now try to imagine the energy required to formulate an idea, to realise a dream etc. One task will be easier for you than the other depending on your predisposition to either the left brain – visual type – or the right brain – auditory type!

Angel advice

Our reaction to people is a direct result of the interconnection between the energy radiating from each person and we will pick up on the 'vibes' (vibrations of energy) of a person depending on our types.

Fascinating Fact

People often refer to the special bond that exists between a parent and child. An explanation of this exists in the production of a bond of energy creating an invisible link. The term soul mate also refers to a bond between people that goes beyond the physical.

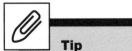

Tip

Homeo = same
Stasis = state.

Energy also flows through the zones, the meridians and the chakras. In a healthy human being, the energy flows freely as all body systems work in harmony with one another creating a state of balance or homeostasis.

It can be said that energy flows through the body with **ease** when a person is well. Energy flow is therefore impeded when the body experiences a state of dis ease. Energy is a source of power that is produced by the interaction of negative and positive polarities and parallels of this theory can be seen in the concept of **yin** and **yang** evolved from traditional Chinese medicine. It describes the theory of a pair of interactive polarities (positive and negative) throughout nature.

Yin and yang

Yin equates to the negative pole and yang the positive pole. The principles of yin and yang are involved with the law of opposites and the idea that a whole is made up of a series of opposites – a back and a front, an exterior and an interior etc. In other words, you cannot have one without the other.

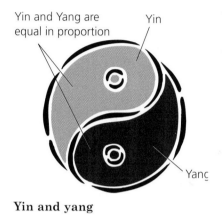

Yin and Yang are equal in proportion

Yin

Yang

Yin and yang

- Yin is also referred to as the female and inactive polarity and is linked to the right brain and auditory types.
- Yang is also referred to as the male and active polarity and is linked to the left brain and visual types.

Good health depends on balance between the two forces.

In life imbalance often forms between these opposites and can result in physical, emotional and spiritual distress. Imbalance affects the flow of energy; thus an awareness of the left and right brain, visual and auditory and yin and yang principles in terms of reflexology provide a basis for rebalance and healing.

Attitudes

There has been a gradual change in the attitudes towards reflexology in the West over recent years. Pioneers of the treatment such as Eunice Ingham and her contemporaries struggled to gain acceptance of the treatment in the twentieth century. Today it is being used with increasing popularity as complementary health practices gain wider acceptance. Evidence of this can be seen throughout all walks of life and across the professions as reflexology is being used with success. Examples include:

- Stress management.
- Management of pain.
- Restoring the quality of life for the terminally ill and their families.
- Aid problems associated with fertility.
- Help with rehabilitation in cases of drug and alcohol dependency.
- Assisting athletes in gaining their competitive edge.

Cultural integration has helped to change attitudes as more and more people accept the different theories associated with health and well-being. This sharing approach enables us to take advantage of all aspects of healing and adapt them to suit individual needs.

Knowledge review

1   How many longitudinal zones apply to reflexology?

2   How many main meridians exist in traditional Chinese medicine and Japanese shiatsu?

3   How many main chakras exist according to Ayurvedic medicine?

4   Visual and auditory types are associated with which sides of the brain?

5   Which type responds more readily to sound and which to visual images and colour?

6   Which side of the brain controls the left side of the body?

7   Which sides of the brain are associated with yin and yang?

8   What do the abbreviations UEF and HEF stand for?

9   What is the definition of homeostasis?

10 What images may be picked up using Kirlian photography?

Methods and practices

3

Methods

Because of the historical background, the resulting theories and changes in attitude, reflexology continues to develop with many variations of the treatment emerging. Reflexology may be applied to the feet, hands and ears and incorporate the specific theories associated with zones, meridians and chakras, colour and sound therapies as well as **visualisations**, **affirmations** and **mantras**.

Feet

Traditionally the feet have provided greatest access to the rest of the body due to their location, size and shape.

- The client is usually seated or lying down for treatment with their feet raised, making this a comfortable position for treatment to take place.
- In recent years vertical reflexology has developed. The client remains in a standing position and all the reflexes are worked from the top of the feet, providing an alternative form of treatment.

Hands

Hands are easily accessible and provide an alternative area for treatment on a number of occasions:

- If the lower limbs have been amputated the zones and reflexes can be easily accessed on the hands.
- If the feet are contraindicated to treatment e.g. painful, infected, inflamed etc. the hands provide the perfect alternative site for treatment.

- The hands also provide easier access for self-treatment.
- The hands and feet may be used in the same treatment.

Ears

The ears are often neglected in terms of general beauty or holistic treatments although they are becoming a more frequent area of focus as treatments such as thermal auricular therapy and Indian head massage are gaining in popularity.

- Reflex points are less accessible due to the size of the ears and the comparative size of the fingers and thumbs.
- Ears provide a good site for self-treatment.
- Ears may be treated prior to or instead of the hands or feet.

Zones

Modern reflexology works on the basis of the zone theory. There are ten longitudinal zones, five on each side of the body, arranged as follows:

- Zone one – extends from the tip of both thumbs up to the top of the head and down through the nostrils to the tip of the big toes.
- Zone two – extends from the tip of the index finger to the head and down to the tip of the second toes.
- Zone three – extends from the tip of the second fingers to the head and down to the tip of the third toes.
- Zone four – extends from the tip of the ring fingers to the head and down to the tip of the fourth toes.
- Zone five – extends from the tip of the little fingers to the head and down to the tip of the little toes.

The body systems, organs and glands can then be mapped out within the appropriate zones.

The body is a macrocosm that is reflected in a microcosm such as the feet, hands and ears (see the colour illustrations of feet, hands and ears at the back of the book).

Angel advice

It is necessary to have a working knowledge of the human body in order to visualise the position of the organs on the hands, feet or ears.

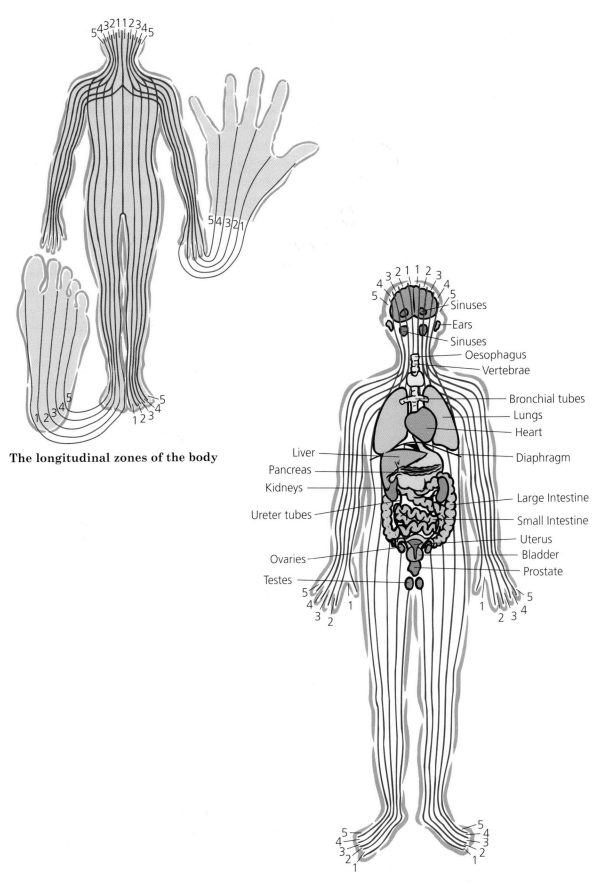

54321 1 2345

543 21

5432 1

5
4 3 2 1

5
4 3 2 1

The longitudinal zones of the body

3 2 1 1 2 3
4 4
5 5

— Sinuses
— Ears
— Sinuses
— Oesophagus
— Vertebrae

— Bronchial tubes
— Lungs
— Heart

Liver —
Pancreas —
Kidneys —

Ureter tubes —

Ovaries —

Testes —

— Diaphragm

— Large Intestine

— Small Intestine
— Uterus
— Bladder
— Prostate

5
4 1
3 2

1 5
2 3 4

5
4
3 2
1

5
4
3 2
1

The body map

Meridians

Traditional Chinese medicine works on the basis of one main channel of energy within the body that divides into fourteen main branches. Twelve of these branches or meridians are linked to an organ of the body. In turn each of these twelve meridians is also associated with either yin or yang. The meridians are coupled to form complementary pairs of yin and yang:

- Liver meridian (yin) coupled with the gall bladder meridian (yang).
- Heart meridian (yin) coupled with the small intestine meridian (yang).

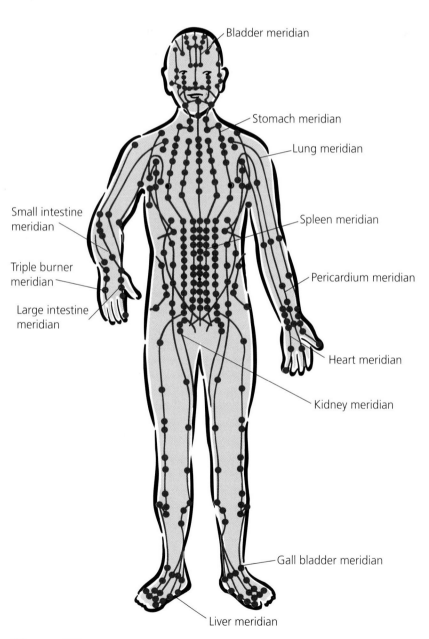

The meridians

- Pericardium (circulation) meridian (yin) coupled with the triple heater (temperature regulation) meridian (yang).
- Kidney meridian (yin) coupled with the bladder meridian (yang).
- Lung meridian (yin) coupled with the large intestine meridian (yang).
- Spleen/pancreas meridian (yin) coupled with the stomach meridian (yang).

These meridians are bilateral, resulting in 24 separate pathways through which energy flows in a twenty-four hour cycle that divides night from day. It is believed that the energy surges into each meridian in two-hourly periods making the corresponding organs more active at that time. The complementary meridians and corresponding organs will be less active during the same time as a result.

The remaining two branches form vessels known as the **conception** and **governing vessels**:

- The conception vessel monitors, regulates and directs the yin meridians (plus the stomach meridian) and is able to increase the yin energy of the body. It is responsible for controlling the life cycle and the changes that occur in a female every seven years and in a male every eight years.
- The governing vessel 'governs' the yang meridians and has a controlling influence on the energy flow within these channels. Because of its position it also controls the back aiding energy flow in this area, which has the effect of guarding the body against 'external evil intruders'.

The energy flows from the earth in an upward direction in the yin meridians and from the sun in a downward direction in the yang meridians, forming a continuous flow or cycle with no beginning or end. The flow moves from the torso to the fingertips to the face and

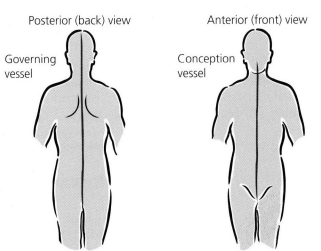

The vessels

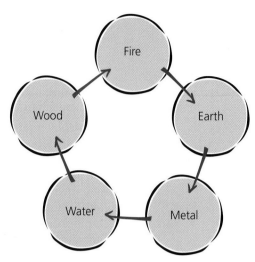

The cycle of elements

to the feet before returning to the torso. The Chinese believe that this cycle of energy is also associated with five elements which form a cycle of their own; **wood**, **fire**, **earth**, **metal** and **water**.

- Wood feeds the fire – wood is needed to create fire.
- Fire feeds the earth – through combustion fire produces organic matter which enriches the soil.
- Earth feeds the metal – the earth produces ores that in turn produce metals.
- Metal feeds the water – minerals dissolve to enrich water.
- Water feeds the wood – water allows trees to grow.

Each element is related to corresponding yin and yang meridians and their associated organs and systems of the body:

- Wood – liver (yin) and gall bladder (yang), muscular and lymphatic systems.
- Fire – heart (yin) and small intestine (yang), cardiovascular and reproductive systems.
- Earth – spleen (yin) and stomach (yang) and nervous and digestive systems.
- Metal – lungs (yin) and large intestine (yang) and the respiratory system.
- Water – kidneys (yin) and bladder (yang) and the skeletal, urinary and endocrine systems.

Fascinating Fact

Metal and water are predominantly associated with yin, right brain and auditory types with wood and fire being predominantly associated with yang, left brain and visual types. Earth is neutral and provides the link between the two.

Chakras

The Ayurvedic medicine of India describes chakras as energy stores, points where the male yang energy and the female yin energy meet. They are situated in line with the spine and can be found on the spinal reflexes of the feet, hands and ears. Chakras

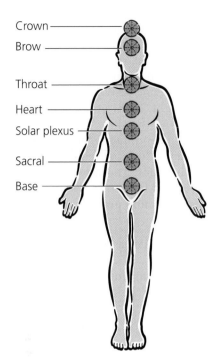

Crown
Brow
Throat
Heart
Solar plexus
Sacral
Base

The chakras

Fascinating Fact

The energy associated with the brow and crown chakras is not earthly and as such is not found in matter.

act as transformers, collecting and storing energy so that it can be used effectively within the body. Like meridians, chakras are also associated with parts of the body and elements, although the elements are classified slightly differently to those associated with the Chinese belief and include ether which represents creation, air, fire, water and earth which are to be found in everything that has been created:

1. Base chakra – all solid parts of the body and the element earth.
2. Sacral chakra – all liquid parts of the body and the element water.
3. Solar plexus chakra – digestive and nervous systems and the element fire.
4. Heart chakra – the cardiovascular system and the element air.
5. Throat chakra – the respiratory system and the element ether.
6. Brow chakra – the central nervous system. There is no associated element.
7. Crown chakra – the central nervous system. There is no associated element.

The chakras are also associated with the endocrine system, with each chakra relating to a specific endocrine gland (see Part 4, Chapter 18 for details).

Colour

The use of colour for healing can be traced back through many civilisations, for example:

●   The early Egyptians built healing temples that were lavishly decorated with colours that radiated healing energy. They also believed that wearing coloured gemstones stopped loss of energy.

●   The ancient Greeks connected colour with healing and linked the colour of body fluids with associated organs e.g. red blood and the heart.

●   In ancient times the Ayurvedic system of India employed the use of colour for all aspects of healing. They worked with minerals and gemstones believing that the frequency of each colour affected the frequencies of the human being.

Medical advancement in the modern world overshadowed the use of colour for healing, but studies and practice now show its beneficial effects when used either as a treatment in its own right or combined with other treatments such as reflexology. Colour is a necessary part of all life. Each living cell is dependent on light for its survival and colour is contained within light. Changes in light affect changes within the body e.g. the sunrise sets off a process within the body that awakens us; sunset and the resulting loss of light sets off another set of processes within the body that induces sleep. The colours contained in light are both visible and invisible with the visible colours making up approximately 40 per cent of the rays of light. The visible colours include red, orange, yellow, green, blue, indigo and violet and can be seen because of their differing frequencies, vibrations and wavelengths. When these colours merge together they form white light. Light enters the body through the sensory organs i.e. the eyes and the skin. The eyes are stimulated by the light entering them and send messages to the brain, which in turn interprets the colours. The skin 'feels' the different vibrations associated with each colour. These processes are mostly unconscious but can be developed for use in treating physical, emotional and spiritual imbalances and are referred to as colour therapy.

Each colour is associated with a meridian and/or a chakra.

- Red – the heart, small intestine, pericardium and triple heater meridians and the base or first chakra.
- Orange – the sacral or second chakra.
- Yellow – the spleen/pancreas and stomach meridians and the solar plexus or third chakra.
- Green – the liver and gall bladder meridians and the heart or fourth chakra.
- Blue – the kidney and bladder meridians and the throat or fifth chakra.
- Indigo – the brow or sixth chakra.
- Violet – the crown or seventh chakra.
- White – the lung and large intestine meridians and the crown or seventh chakra.

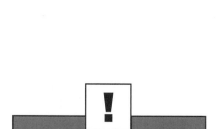

Remember

The left brain visual types respond more readily to the use of colour.

Angel advice

Colour may be used in the treatment room with the use of decoration, pictures, towels and blankets etc. I like to have various objects such as angels and fairies of different colours in my treatment room. My clients tend to home in on a particular object and the associated colour depending on their needs without even realising it. In addition, I find that I am instinctively drawn towards the use of a particular colour towel for each treatment.

Sound

Sound is carried by vibration and can be used in combination with pressure to each part of the body or reflex point, providing the potential for greater effect. Sensitive fingers can pick up on the vibration of each reflex point and apply a corresponding sound either in the form of a musical note or just by saying the notes.

This technique forms the basis for sound therapy. There are seven musical notes – A, B, C, D, E, F and G. Each note is associated with a meridian and/or a chakra:

- A – the liver and small intestine meridians and the brow or sixth chakra.
- B – the crown or seventh chakra.
- C – the heart and lung meridians and the base or first chakra.
- D – the small intestine and bladder meridians and the sacral or second chakra.
- E – the solar plexus or third chakra.
- F – the spleen/pancreas and kidney meridians and the heart or fourth chakra.
- G – the large intestine and gall bladder meridians, the throat or the fifth chakra.

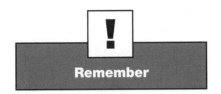

Remember

Right brain auditory types respond more readily to sound.

 Angel advice

It is common practice to play music during a reflexology treatment. The sound is carried by vibrations and picked up both by the client and the practitioner, having an affect on their general well-being. Soothing music will calm our senses, bringing about a feeling of relaxation.

Visualisation

Visualisation is a technique incorporating the conscious use of positive images and/or colour to bring about physiological changes in the body. Visualisation gives people an element of control over their own well-being.

- The practitioner can use visualisations to help with the focus of the treatment.
- The client can be encouraged to help themselves with the use of visualisations to shift their focus from the negative and towards the positive.

Remember

Strong visual images are easily picked up by left brain visual types.

 Angel advice

Cards depicting a positive image may be used at the end of the treatment to encourage further use of visualisation.

Angel advice

For some clients I like to use cards with a positive word printed and a corresponding picture on them at the end of the treatment. I have a basket with 52 cards and ask the client to choose a card at random whilst focusing on an aspect of their well-being that may have been highlighted in the treatment. The spoken word appeals to our right brain auditory type and the picture to the left brain visual type. Using both helps to obtain balance.

Affirmations and mantras

Affirmations involve the use of positive words to voice intent. Words can be expressed as a feeling, out loud or in writing and provide the link between thought and action. Affirmations are a positive focus on an end result.

- The practitioner can use affirmations to focus on the intent of reflexology both at the start and close of the treatment.
- The client can be taught to use affirmations to focus the mind on the intent of the treatment and also as a positive focus at the start and close of each day.

Mantras are special phrases that can be used to focus on the energy flowing within and all around us. Mantras can be used to bring about a state of meditation and are generally said aloud.

The client and practitioner can be encouraged to use a mantra to stimulate individual chakras:

- Lam for the first chakra.
- Vam for the second chakra.
- Ram for the third chakra.
- Yam for the fourth chakra.
- Ham for the fifth chakra.
- Ksham for the sixth chakra.
- Om for the seventh chakra.

Alternatively 'Om', which is a universal mantra meaning 'I am all that which is divine' can be used as a general mantra.

The mantras may be spoken or sung using the corresponding note (see sound on page 26 for corresponding notes) adding to the therapeutic effect of sound therapy.

Practices

Reflexology today is practiced by many people from many walks of life and professions in a variety of places including:

- Salons – an increasing number of beauty salons incorporate reflexology in the services they offer.
- Spas – are becoming a popular venue for relaxing, therapeutic treatments such as reflexology.
- Clinics – practitioners who specialise purely in reflexology may operate out of private clinics.
- Health clubs, centres and hydros – increasing awareness amongst athletes has prompted the use of reflexology in a sports context.

- Home – many people seeking reflexology would prefer to be treated in the comfort of their own home, making it a popular mobile therapy.

- Workplace – many employers are realising the effects of stress on their workforce and the links to absenteeism. Current legislation is forcing employers to take responsibility for the stress levels of their employees, thus workplace treatment is fast becoming a viable option for stress-free work zones.

- Hospitals – reflexology is being used to help in the relief of pain. Particular areas of benefit include during childbirth.

- Addiction clinics – reflexology is being used with increasing success in cases of drug and alcohol addiction. It can be used to balance and maintain a drug/alcohol free state in recovering addicts as well as help in the various stages of becoming drug/alcohol free.

- Mental health – reflexology provides a simple method of effective communication for people of all ages, providing a means of gaining trust and security in a sometimes frightening world.

- General practices and health centres – reflexology is becoming increasingly accepted within the medical profession and is often incorporated in the general facilities offered as part of a programme promoting good health by nurses, midwives, counsellors etc.

- Hospices – the use of reflexology for the terminally ill has proved to be of value to both patients and families.

- Schools – reflexology has been seen to aid disruptive and hyperactive children and many schools will use practitioners of reflexology for help with children with a variety of social problems.

- Nursing homes – the benefit of reflexology for the elderly can be seen in all aspects of an older person's life and is used with increasing popularity.

- Complementary – reflexology is often used as an additional service in establishments that offer osteopathy, physiotherapy, chiropody, homeopathy, acupuncture, iridology, kinesiology, crystal therapy etc.

- Retreats – reflexology is a popular treatment for people seeking personal enlightenment on a physical, emotional and spiritual basis.

Tip

Practitioners of reflexology may choose to call themselves therapists or reflexologists regardless of their background, which may include medical, complementary, sports, beauty or holistic therapy.

Knowledge review

1   Give one reason why the ears are a useful site for the application of reflexology.

2   Name the five elements used in traditional Chinese medicine.

3   How do the elements used in Ayurvedic treatment differ?

4   Name the seven chakras.

5   What are the seven visible colours included in light?

6   What are affirmations?

7   What are visualisations?

8   What are mantras?

9   Give an example of six places of work where reflexology treatment may be practiced.

10   What is the meaning of complementary therapies?

Objectives of reflexology

The general objectives of reflexology can be classified as physical, emotional and spiritual in a quest to gain a greater sense of awareness of the body, mind and spirit in order to restore and maintain balance as well as stimulate the body's own **healing** mechanisms.

The specific outcomes of a single treatment or a course of treatments may be a result of a stronger focus on one or other of the general objectives, depending on the needs of the client and the skills of the practitioner.

Physical

The focus of treatment on the physical is a good starting point for both the client and the practitioner. A person may be alerted to the fact that all is not well by the physical symptoms they are experiencing. Focusing on the physical helps to create greater self-awareness and encourage a person to take more responsibility for their own well-being by listening to what their body needs and responding with the appropriate action.

Emotional

The links between emotional and physical symptoms can be a further focus for treatment, providing greater potential for future well-being. By focusing on the way in which our emotions affect our physical well-being and vice versa, self-awareness increases and self-development begins to take place.

Spiritual

A natural progression for clients and practitioners is to realise the intrinsic bond that links a person to everything that is around them. This recognition enables the treatment to reach the next level in terms of drawing on the healing powers of the universe and their associated energies.

Awareness

Reflexology is all about learning for both practitioners and clients. As we learn about the treatment we discover more about our clients and ourselves. As we progress with the treatment experiential learning broadens this knowledge. Having an inquisitive and open mind encourages us to take on board and further develop the various theories as well as formulate those of our own, and put into practice only those that we feel comfortable with, being aware that as we change so does the treatment we perform and receive.

Balance

Balancing or 'bringing about a state of equilibrium' is a term often used to describe the objectives of reflexology. The history and resulting theories emerging from the various cultures all lead us in a similar direction towards the Eastern paradigm of creating a dynamic state of balance and the Western criterion of achieving homeostasis. Each of the methods discussed in this part can be applied as a means of balancing the body, mind and spirit. Incorporating a mix of methods may further enhance this balancing act. Adaptations of the treatment may be explored practically and intuitively in order to perform the treatment suited to your clients' needs at any given time.

Angel advice

Learn the theory to develop your left brain activity; experience the practice to develop your right brain activity – and become a well-balanced practitioner.

Healing

The definition of healing is 'to make or become well'. It can also be described as the process of returning to normal or *ease* of function after a period of *dis ease*. Reflexology and its associated methods of treatment aims to activate the body's own healing mechanisms. This does not mean that it provides a cure; rather that it provides an holistic approach to 'becoming well' and should be seen as being complementary to many other methods including those which are more and indeed less conventional e.g.

- As a doctor or nurse studying reflexology we may incorporate our medical knowledge and skill to 'heal' the patient.
- As a practitioner of reiki studying reflexology, we may incorporate our ability to channel energy to 'heal' the client.

It is important to be aware of the process of healing and how as part of this process some clients may experience a 'healing reaction'. Treatments such as reflexology aim to stimulate the body's own healing mechanisms which initiates a set of reactions that force the body to give in to its own needs (rather like the reaction a person may experience when they allow themselves to relax). This may mean that the person needs to give in to the physical and/or emotional reactions – tiredness, tearfulness etc. – or even the illness they have been fighting off as they begin to experience the symptoms post-treatment. The treatment has not made them tired, weepy or ill; their body has forced them to be more aware and to feel the associated symptoms. The balancing effects of the treatment will help the body to deal with the symptoms more effectively in the short term and further treatments, together with medical treatment if necessary, will give more long-term benefits. Continued treatment will ensure that the body functions at its best and help to prevent problems in the future.

A–Z of complementary therapies

With these objectives in mind, here are many treatments that can be used with and/or along side reflexology including:

- ACUPRESSURE – involves the use of finger pressure on acupuncture points throughout the body to stimulate the flow of energy. It is similar to shiatsu.
- ACUPUNCTURE – the Chinese practice of inserting fine needles along points of the meridians where energy has become blocked to aid in the relief of pain and to improve the natural healing mechanisms of the body.
- ALEXANDER TECHNIQUE – the correction of poor posture and body alignment to relieve associated problems. It involves a process of re-education to restore harmony within the body as a whole.
- AROMATHERAPY – the use of essential oils from flowers, herbs, trees, resins and spices to treat the body, mind and spirit. The oils can be used in a variety of ways to enhance well-being and improve general health. They can be diluted in a carrier oil and applied directly onto the skin during massage, used in diffusers and vaporisers, inhaled directly, diluted in baths, used in compresses and applied neat.
- AURICULAR THERAPY/AURICULOTHERAPY – stimulation of the ear by pressure from fingers, needles and/or instruments to release energy and work specific reflex points.
- AUTOGENIC TRAINING – a system of six standard self-help exercises which induce a state of deep relaxation. The techniques teach the art of passive concentration which in turn improves communication between the left and right hemispheres of the brain bringing about a more balanced interaction of the body as a whole.
- AYURVEDA – a traditional Indian form of healing. It can be translated as 'ayus' meaning 'life' and 'veda'

meaning science or knowledge. Ayurveda therefore incorporates the knowledge of a whole lifestyle to bring about healing. It works on the assumption that everything is made up of five basic elements – fire, water, earth, air and ether – and that people have dominant characteristics – pitta, kapha and vata – that are prone to certain diseases and so can be treated according to their needs.

- BACH FLOWER REMEDIES – remedies formulated from flowers and trees that have a positive effect on the negative emotions often associated with disease. There are 38 different remedies that treat problems associated with emotional loss of control such as depression, fear and anxiety.

- BOWEN TECHNIQUE – developed in Australia, it is a method of rebalancing the flow of energy throughout the body with the use of light rolling manual techniques over the muscles.

- CHINESE HERBAL MEDICINE – forms part of the ancient system of traditional Chinese medicine (TCM). According to Chinese herbal medicine herbs have five flavours, five energy (chi) characteristics and four directions. These factors are all considered in the preparation of a formula, which may be prescribed as a healing remedy.

- CHIROPRACTIC – from the Greek words *cheir* meaning 'hand' and *praktikos* meaning 'done by'. Manipulations are used to treat mechanical problems that arise in the joints of the body to relieve pain, improve function and mobility. This has the effect of re-establishing the relationship between the spinal column and the musculo-skeletal system helping the whole body function more efficiently as one. It is similar to osteopathy but the focus is mainly on the spine and its effects on the nervous system.

- COLOUR THERAPY – the use of varied frequencies associated with different colours to balance the frequency within the body. The cells of a healthy body vibrate at a constant frequency. Ill-health creates inconsistent frequencies that can be restored by introducing the vibration of colours through sight, touch and/or visualisation. Colour therapy is often used with other treatments such as reflexology.

- COUNSELLING – a means of talking through a problem with a counsellor to build better coping mechanisms.

- CRYSTAL THERAPY – crystals and gemstones generate, store and give off energies that match those of the body, mind and spirit. Used on and around the body they can bring about a healing and balancing effect.

- CYMATICS – from the Greek word *kyma* meaning 'a great wave', cymatics is a form of sound therapy. Specialised machinery is used to create sound waves that operate on the same level as healthy cells. When used on a body that is injured or diseased this has the effect of rebalancing energy and restoring health.

- DAOYIN TAO – Chinese face, neck and shoulder massage. A combination of ancient Chinese and modern Western massage techniques.

- FENG SHUI – ancient Oriental system of organising a place of work or a home in such a way as to encourage a free flow of energy which in turn promotes greater health, wealth and happiness.

- GONG THERAPY – a sonic massage is created through the sound produced when a gong is struck at a predetermined pitch. The rhythm and intensity of the resulting sound stimulates and balances energy flow to induce relaxation and well-being.

- HERBAL MEDICINE – the original medicine formulated from the healing properties of plants to treat disease.

- HOMEOPATHY – originating from the Greek word *homios* meaning 'like' and *pathos* meaning 'suffering'. The treatment works on the law of similars i.e. 'that which makes sick shall heal'. Ingredients are formulated from plants and minerals to form a remedy that if used in large doses would cause a set of symptoms of illness in a healthy person. When used in minute doses the same remedy would act as an aid to similar symptoms experienced in a sick person.

- HYPNOTHERAPY – an altered state of consciousness is induced through deep relaxation and is able to bring about the relief of physical, emotional and spiritual problems.

- IRIDOLOGY – a diagnostic therapy incorporating the eyes. The iris of the eye can be divided into twelve segments that reflect the whole of the body. Changes detected within these segments relate directly to corresponding organs and systems of the body as a whole.

- KINESIOLOGY – taken from the Greek words *kinesis* meaning 'movement' and *ology* meaning 'study of'. A process of muscle testing to determine areas of the body that have suffered a block in energy flow. Energy flow can be restored by an increase in muscle strength.

- MASSAGE – the use of pressure techniques to promote a feeling of well-being incorporating the use of effleurage (stroking), petrissage (deep) and tapotement (stimulating) movements.

- MEDITATION – a technique based on reflection and contemplation for attaining a state of relaxation in order to calm the body, mind and spirit. The use of mantras or special phrases helps to focus the mind and allow the energy to flow freely.

- METAMORPHIC TECHNIQUE – a form of manipulation therapy similar to that of reflexology that has the effect of stimulating energy. The spinal reflexes are worked on the feet, hands and head relating to stages in a person's life from conception onwards to bring about an emotional, behavioural and/or physical transformation.

- NATUROPATHY – the coordination of natural resources to restore and maintain perfect health. Resources include air, water, whole foods, sunlight, relaxation and exercise. It is a lifestyle method that focuses on the whole body.

- NUTRITIONAL THERAPY – a method of stimulating healing by means of a balanced intake of food and nutrition.

- OSTEOPATHY – a system of therapy based on the manipulation of the body's structure to relieve pain, improve mobility and restore general health. Cranial osteopathy uses specialist techniques to manipulate the bones of the skull to balance the cerebrospinal fluid that in turn stimulates the body's own healing mechanisms.

- PAST LIFE THERAPY – a method of regression guiding a person back in time to another life in order to discover and heal the causes of physical and/or emotional difficulties experienced in their current life.

- PHYSIOTHERAPY – the application of massage and the use of exercise to re-establish the use of the musculo-skeletal system in cases of illness, injury and/or surgery.

- POLARITY THERAPY – is the science of balancing the electromagnetic energy that flows between negative and positive poles. It incorporates both Western and Eastern theories of healing to unblock energy with the use of four techniques – touch, awareness skills, diet and exercise.

- PILATES – a fusion of Eastern and Western philosophies producing a set of exercises similar to yoga that work the body as a whole to improve flexibility, strength, posture and coordination. The basic principles include: centring, alignment, breathing, control, precision, flowing movement and relaxation.

- RADIONICS – the use of specialist instruments to analyse illness and energy imbalance. The analysis is usually of a strand of hair, but may be of a drop of blood or a nail clipping which provides a link to the state of an individual's energy field. As a result of the analysis complementary treatments may be prescribed.

- REIKI – reiki comes from the Japanese words *rei* meaning 'universal' and *ki* meaning 'energy'. It incorporates a technique that works on balancing energy flow to aid healing. There are three stages to reiki: *reiki 1* teaches the practitioner to use the energy on themselves, their friends, families and pets as well as plants and food. *Reiki 2* takes the principles a stage further with the use of ancient symbols that activate the use of energy to greater benefit and may be used on clients. *Reiki master* allows the teaching of reiki to be passed from a Master to a layperson.

- ROLFING – a method of re-aligning the body's structure through manipulation. By using the fingertips, hands and knuckles this has the overall effect of realigning the body with the forces of gravity enabling the body to heal itself more efficiently and effectively. HELLERWORK is a derivative of rolfing and works on the same basic principles.

- SHIATSU – originates from Japan and involves the treatment of the body, mind and spirit through massage. Pressure is applied to the *tsubo* points along the meridians by either the fingers, palms, elbows, arms, knees and/or feet. This has the effect of freeing blocked energy within the meridians.

- SOUND THERAPY – the use of sound to rebalance the frequencies associated with illness. Sound may be in the form of a specific note or by use of the letter associated with the sound e.g. A, B, C etc.

- SPIRITUAL HEALING – a means of channelling energy to bring about a sense of well-being and to encourage healing.

- T'AI CHI – meaning 'supreme unity' it is an ancient Chinese method of exercise that works on the flow of energy to improve health and well-being. It has developed into a non-violent martial art.

- THERMAL AURICULAR THERAPY – a traditional Native American therapy for the treatment of ears to unblock excessive mucus congestion, helping to free the energy and clear the mind. The treatment incorporates the use of specialised candles that work on a 'chimney' principal gently clearing the ears and associated regions e.g. sinuses, nose and throat. A safe and effective alternative to the Western method of syringing the ears.

- TRADITIONAL CHINESE MEDICINE (TCM) – a complete system of healing developed by the ancient Chinese based on the system of meridians and the flow of chi.

- WESTERN HERBALISM – the traditional use of plants as medicines combined with modern scientific developments to restore and maintain general health and well-being.

- YOGA – a non-competitive form of exercise that incorporates a set of postures or 'asanas' and breathing techniques or 'pranayamas' to improve the flow of energy or 'prana' around the body. This has a calming, restoring and strengthening effect on the body, mind and spirit.

- ZONE THERAPY – the application of pressure at a point within the zone or pathway to stimulate the flow of energy in the whole zone. Extreme pressure may be used as a means of blocking extreme pain.

Task

Choose five of the complementary therapies listed in the A–Z.

Using whatever resources are available to you, complete further research on each one. Include in your research the following information:

- History of the treatment
- Effect and benefits
- Contraindications
- Application of the treatment.

Tip

A good way of researching a treatment is to find a local practitioner and book an appointment for a treatment. Alternatively try to attend local complementary therapy/health fairs where practitioners are available to discuss their therapies in more detail. In addition, the Internet provides a wealth of information.

Part 2

The skills

Learning objectives

After reading this chapter you should be able to:

- **Recognise the structure of the feet, hands and ears.**

- **Identify the skills needed to practice reflexology.**

- **Understand the functions of the feet, hands and ears.**

- **Be aware of links between the theoretical, practical and psychological skills.**

- **Begin to appreciate the ways in which the skills contribute to the treatment.**

Reflexology is a treatment that deals with the whole of a human being through a part i.e. the feet, hands and/or ears. As a result, it is important for the practitioner to have acquired a set of skills that enable them to carry out a safe and successful treatment. These skills can be categorised as being theoretical, practical and psychological and may be linked with the mind, body and spirit.

Theoretical skills

5

One of the most important tools for a practitioner of reflexology is having a working knowledge of the **anatomy** and **physiology** of the whole body, because the theory relating to the structure and function of the parts forms the basis of the treatment. An understanding of the **terms of reference** enables us to identify areas for treatment and a working knowledge of the **common conditions** affecting the parts provides us with the means to determine whether or not it is a suitable area for treatment.

Anatomy and physiology

Tip

Anatomy refers to the *structure* of the body whilst physiology refers to the *function* of the body.

The human body is made up of millions and millions of individual microscopic cells.

Fascinating Fact

Cells provide the building blocks with which the human body is formed.

Groups of cells form the four types of tissue:

- Epithelial tissue for protection e.g. skin, linings and coverings of vessels and organs.

- Connective tissue for support e.g. areolar, adipose, lymphoid, elastic, fibrous, cartilage, bone and blood.
- Muscular tissue for movement e.g. skeletal, visceral and cardiac.
- Nervous tissue for sensation e.g. neurons and neuroglia.

Different types of tissue are joined together to form organs and glands:

- Organs have a specific structure and function and consist of two or more tissue types e.g. brain, heart, liver, lungs, stomach etc.
- Glands are formed from epithelial tissue and produce specialised substances. Endocrine glands produce hormones and exocrine glands produce substances such as sebum and sweat.

Remember

Endocrine glands are ductless glands passing their substances directly into the bloodstream. Exocrine glands pass their substances into ducts e.g. sebaceous glands pass sebum into the hair follicle.

Groups of associated organs and glands that have a common function form body systems i.e. integumentary, skeletal, muscular, respiratory, circulatory, digestive, genito-urinary, nervous and endocrine systems.

System overview

Integumentary system – consisting of the skin, hair and nails. This system provides the body with a waterproof protective outer covering that is resilient, flexible and contributes to our unique personal appearance.

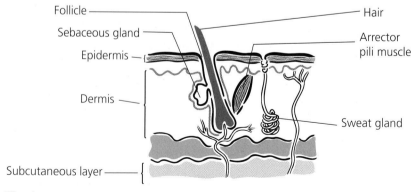

The integumentary system

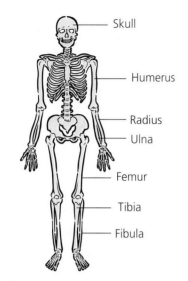

Skull

Humerus

Radius

Ulna

Femur

Tibia

Fibula

The skeletal system

Skeletal system – consisting of 206 individual bones with the formation of joints supported by cartilage and ligaments. This system provides the body with a framework that is solid in structure and flexible in function.

Muscular system – consisting of skeletal, visceral and cardiac muscular tissue and responsible for voluntary and involuntary movement. Muscles function like motors by producing the force to make a movement of the external and internal parts of the body.

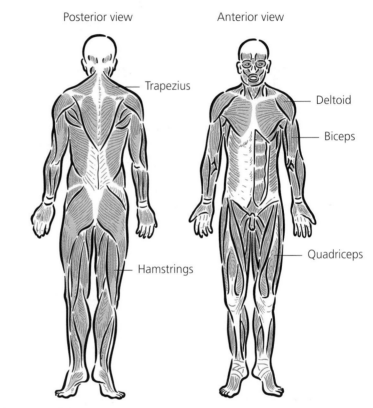

Posterior view

Anterior view

Trapezius

Deltoid

Biceps

Hamstrings

Quadriceps

The muscular system

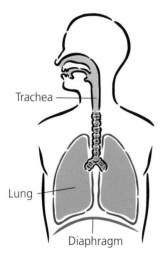

Trachea

Lung

Diaphragm

The respiratory system

Respiratory system – consisting of external openings into the body, i.e. the nose and mouth, together with a network of air passageways leading to the lungs. The respiratory system is responsible for breathing oxygen into the body and carbon dioxide out of the body i.e. respiration.

Circulatory systems – consisting of two complementary systems – blood circulation and lymphatic circulation – which work together to provide the body with a transportation network for the supply of nourishment, e.g. nutrients and oxygen, and the removal of waste, e.g. carbon dioxide etc.

Digestive system – starts at the mouth extending down into the area of the trunk below the diaphragm and consists of the alimentary canal together with the accessory organs (liver, gall bladder and pancreas). It is responsible for supplying the body with vital nutrients for growth, maintenance and general well-being.

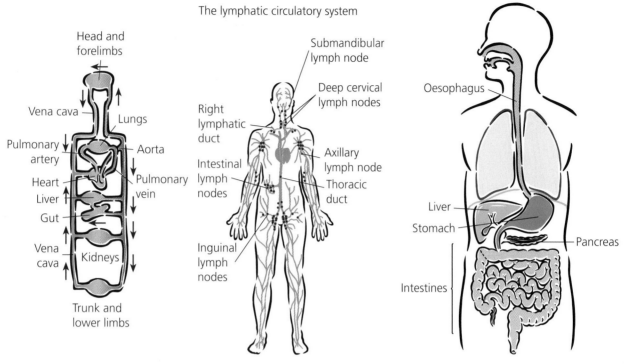

The lymphatic circulatory system

The circulatory systems

The digestive system

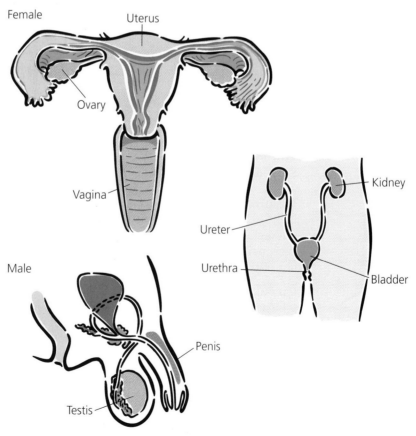

The genito-urinary system

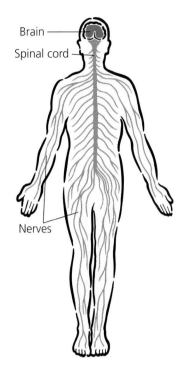

Brain
Spinal cord
Nerves

The nervous system

Genito-urinary system – two closely linked systems; the genitalia responsible for reproduction and the urinary organs responsible for the elimination of excess water and waste from the body.

Nervous system – a complex communication system that allows the body to detect external and internal changes through the sensory organs and to make use of the information received to form a response by stimulating the muscles and organs into action. Consists of the central, peripheral and autonomic nervous systems.

Endocrine system – closely linked to the nervous system, the endocrine system communicates with chemical messengers or hormones. Hormones are produced in endocrine glands and pass directly into the bloodstream to be transported to the part of the body they are to communicate with.

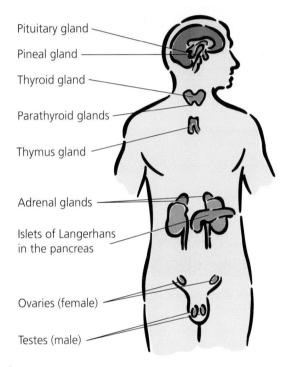

Pituitary gland
Pineal gland
Thyroid gland
Parathyroid glands
Thymus gland
Adrenal glands
Islets of Langerhans in the pancreas
Ovaries (female)
Testes (male)

The endocrine system

An organism is formed as all the body systems function with one another, producing a living human being. In Part 4 the systems of the body are discussed in more detail and linked to form an appropriate order of work for the application of reflexology treatment.

Our feet, hands and ears all form points of connection between the whole of a human being and the world around us as well as providing mirror images of the body, mind and spirit within us.

Feet

The feet form the connection point between the body and the earth we stand upon and, through reflexology treatment, provide the greatest access to the person that lies within us.

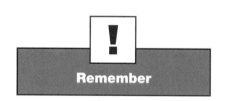

Structure and function

The feet are made up of skin, bones and muscles and are linked to the rest of the body via the circulatory and nervous systems. Their functions include support and coordinated movement – walking, running, jumping etc.

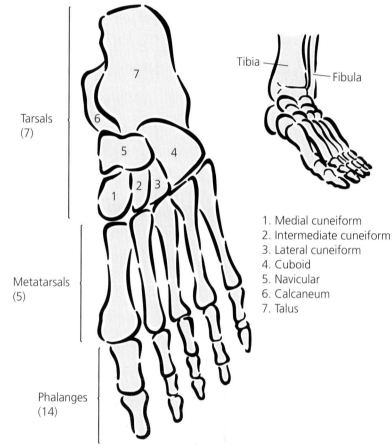

1. Medial cuneiform
2. Intermediate cuneiform
3. Lateral cuneiform
4. Cuboid
5. Navicular
6. Calcaneum
7. Talus

The bones of the lower leg and foot

The feet form part of the appendicular skeleton and include:

- Tarsal bones – seven tarsal bones forming each ankle.
- Metatarsal bones – five metatarsal bones forming the length of each foot.
- Phalange bones – fourteen phalange bones forming the toes of each foot.

Ligaments attach bone to bone at joints, flexor and extensor muscles provide the feet with movement and the muscles of the lower leg provide movement in the ankle. Tendons attach the muscles to the bones: one of the main tendons of the feet is the Achilles tendon.

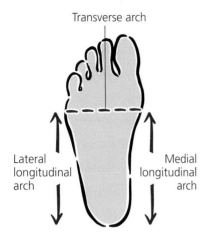

The arches of the feet

The feet have three major arches that distribute the weight of the body between the ball and the heel when the body is standing or walking.

1. Medial longitudinal arch – running along the inside of the feet.
2. Lateral longitudinal arch – running along the outside of the feet.
3. Transverse arch – running across the feet.

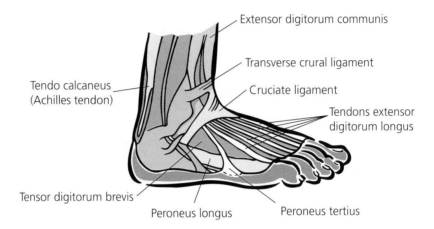

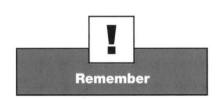

Remember

The bones of the feet, the ligaments connecting them and the muscles of the feet maintain the shape of the arches.

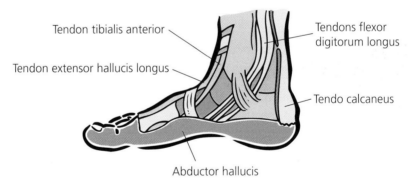

The muscles and tendons of the foot

Hands

The hands form the first physical connection point between people and as such provide an invaluable tool for the giving and receiving of reflexology treatment.

Structure and function

The hands are made up of skin, bones and muscles and like the feet are linked to the rest of the body via the circulatory and nervous systems. Their functions include support and coordinated movement – holding, lifting, picking up etc.

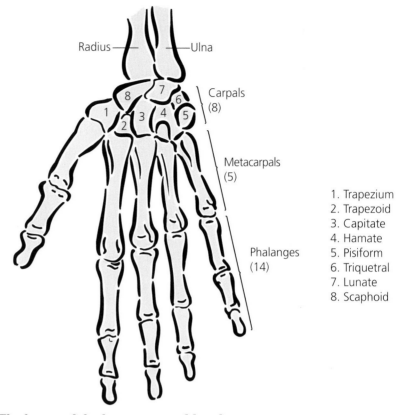

The bones of the lower arm and hand

1. Trapezium
2. Trapezoid
3. Capitate
4. Hamate
5. Pisiform
6. Triquetral
7. Lunate
8. Scaphoid

The hands form part of the appendicular skeleton and include:

● Carpal bones – eight carpal bones forming each wrist.
● Metacarpal bones – five metacarpal bones forming the palm of each hand.

Remember

Each finger and thumb has a nail that provides added protection to the tip.

Remember

The hands are attached at the wrist to the ulna and radius bones of the forearm.

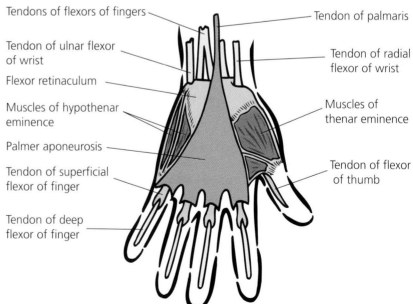

The muscles and tendons of the hand

Remember

The joints between these bones form synovial (freely moveable) joints.

- Phalange bones – fourteen phalange bones forming the fingers and thumb of each hand.

Ligaments attach the bones at joints, flexor and extensor muscles in the lower arm and hand provide movement in the wrist, hand and fingers and tendons attach these muscles to the bones.

Ears

The ears form external and internal connection points through the sense of hearing and balance. They also contain an image of the body as a whole and so are suitable for the application of reflexology treatment.

Structure and function

The external portion (outer ear) of the ear or earflap is known as the pinna, the auditory canal and the eardrum. The internal portion of the ear is made up of the middle and inner ear. They are linked to the rest of the body via the circulatory and nervous systems. Several muscles attach to the ear but they remain undeveloped. The ears are associated with the sensory functions of balance and hearing.

The external ear consists of:

- The pinna, also known as the auricle and made up of a lower section or lobule (ear lobe) and an upper section or helix. The lobe is composed of fibrous and adipose tissue and has a rich blood supply. The helix is comprised of fibroelastic cartilage and has a poor blood supply.

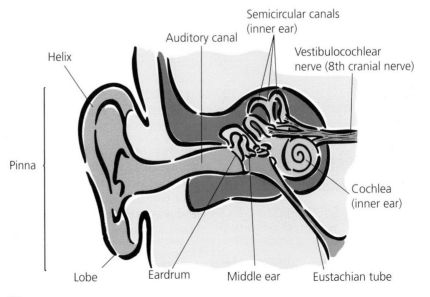

The ear

Remember

The Eustachian tube links the middle ear with the nasopharynx and is responsible for maintaining equal pressure in the eardrum. When there is unequal pressure the Eustachian tube opens and equalises the pressure. Yawning and swallowing opens the Eustachian tube and the equalising of pressure can be experienced as a 'popping' in the ears.

Fascinating Fact

Loss of balance occurs when the brain cannot keep up with the changes in movement of the head e.g. spinning in a circle – this causes us to lose our balance and fall over!

Fascinating Fact

Sound is measured in decibels (dB) and normal conversation would measure approximately 65dB. Sound used during treatment should be at this level or lower so as not to aggravate the ears.

Remember

Sensory nerves transmit impulses *to* the central nervous system and motor nerves transmit impulses *away* from the central nervous system.

- The auditory canal, also known as the external auditory meatus, forms an s-shaped tube approximately 2.5 cm in length extending from the pinna to the eardrum. Fine hairs line the skin of the auditory canal together with glands responsible for the formation of cerumen (earwax), both of these offer a form of protection.
- The eardrum or tympanic membrane is cone-shaped and consists of an outer covering of hairless skin, a middle layer of fibrous tissue and an inner lining of mucous membrane.

The middle ear or tympanic cavity is an irregular-shaped cavity containing three small bones called malleus, incus and stapes, the auditory ossicles which are held in place by fine ligaments and which form a series of moveable joints. The auditory ossicles form a bridge between the eardrum and the inner ear.

The inner ear consists of fluid filled tubes called labyrinths, which form the semicircular canals, responsible for our sense of balance, and the cochlea, which is responsible for our sense of hearing.

The ears detect changes in the position of the head and send messages via the vestibulocochlear eighth cranial nerve to the brain. The messages are interpreted and the skeletal muscles are instructed to maintain posture and thus balance.

Sound waves are picked up by the pinna and directed into the auditory canal to the eardrum where they pass through the middle ear to the inner ear, are picked up by the cochlea and transmitted to the brain via the vestibulocochlear eighth cranial nerve for interpretation.

The feet, hands and ears are all linked to the rest of the body through the circulatory and nervous systems. The circulatory systems provide nourishment, e.g. oxygen and nutrients, via arteries (the blood circulation) and aid in the removal of waste products, e.g. carbon dioxide etc., via veins and lymphatic vessels (blood and lymph circulation).

The cranial and spinal nerves of the peripheral nervous system link the parts of the body to the central nervous system (spinal cord and brain) allowing the integration, translation and storage of feelings and responses via sensory and motor nerves.

Terms of reference

These are used to identify the various anatomical positions or aspects. The anatomical terms of reference applicable to reflexology include:

- Anterior – front
- Posterior – back
- Dorsal – the posterior surface
- Plantar – the sole or underside of the foot (anterior surface)
- Palmar – the palm or underside of the hand (anterior surface)
- Midline – the line through the centre of the body
- Median – the centre
- Medial – towards the midline
- Lateral – away from the midline
- Longitudinal – running from top to bottom
- Transverse – running across
- Distal – the furthest point away from an attachment
- Proximal – the closest point to an attachment.

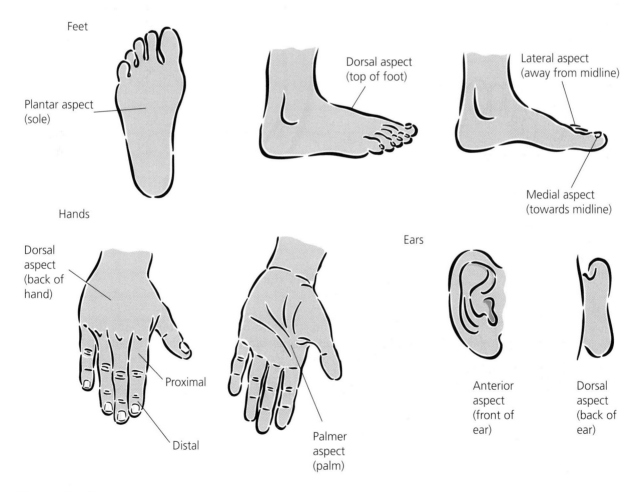

Feet

Plantar aspect (sole)

Dorsal aspect (top of foot)

Lateral aspect (away from midline)

Medial aspect (towards midline)

Hands

Dorsal aspect (back of hand)

Proximal

Distal

Palmer aspect (palm)

Ears

Anterior aspect (front of ear)

Dorsal aspect (back of ear)

Terms of reference specific to the ears include:

- Lobe – ear lobe
- Helix – the outer rim of the auricle of the ear
- Antihelix – the semicircular ridge on the flap of the ear
- Fossa – a small depression or dip
- Concha – the hollow of the auricle
- Tragus – the cartilaginous projection in front of the external opening of the ear
- Antitragus – a projection on the ear opposite to the tragus
- Scapha – the curved depression separating the helix and antihelix.

Feet

Shoulder line

Diaphragm line

Waist line

Pelvic line

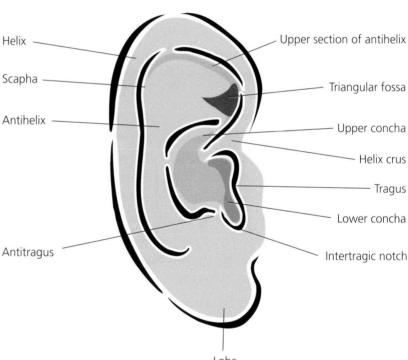

Terms of reference for the ear

Hands

Shoulder line

Diaphragm line

Waist line

Pelvic line

Dividing lines on the feet and hands

The feet and hands can also be divided into sections that correspond with the lines of the body in the following way:

- Shoulder line
- Diaphragm line
- Waist line
- Pelvic line.

These terms of reference provide the reflexology practitioner with the means to 'map out' the whole of the human body on one of its parts (see the colour illustrations at the back of the book).

Common conditions

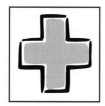

Holistic practitioners believe that the whole body cannot be well unless all of its parts are well. However, when carrying out a reflexology treatment it is important to recognise conditions that can affect the feet, hands and ears including those that may be made worse by treating the part or result in possible cross-infection i.e. contraindications.

Conditions that lead to disease and illness are the result of a break down of cells and may be caused by a number of factors including: genetic e.g. inherited conditions, degenerative e.g. ageing, environmental or chemical, and microbes e.g. viruses, bacteria, fungi and parasites. In some cases genetic and degenerative conditions may be aggravated by treatment and microbes are infectious and may be passed from person to person during treatment.

A–Z of disorders and diseases affecting the feet, hands and ears

Angel advice

If you are likely to cause cross-infection by working over an area it is contra indicated to treatment. Treat an alternative site.

- ACROCYANOSIS – poor circulation of the hands, fingers, feet and toes. A harmless but persistent condition associated with young women.
- ACROMEGALY – abnormal enlargement of the feet, hands and face accompanied by thickening of the skin caused by overproduction of the growth hormone by the pituitary gland.
- ACROPARAESTHESIA – intense tingling or prickly sensation in the fingers or the toes. May be caused by pressure on a nerve. More common in women, it is thought to be associated with the chemical changes in the body caused by menstruation. May also be associated with Raynaud's syndrome.
- ARTHRITIS – a general term for the inflammation of a joint.
- ATHLETE'S FOOT – a fungal infection, also known as tinea pedis, which is a form of ringworm. Most common on the soles of the feet and in between the toes. Symptoms include itchy, soggy, flaking and peeling skin.
- BLISTER – a swelling formed by a build up of fluid under the skin. Often found on the feet as a result of new or ill-fitting shoes.
- BRITTLE NAILS (fragilitas unguium) – excessively dry nails.
- BUERGER'S DISEASE – progressive destruction of the blood vessels in the feet and sometimes the hands. Symptoms include pain, discolouration, numbness, burning and/or tingling and the area feels cold. It can be associated with heavy smoking.

- BUNION (hallux valgus) – harmless swelling of the joint of the big toe. The big toe bends towards the other toes and the skin becomes hard, red and tender.
- BURSITIS – inflammation of the bursa (a sac-like extension of the synovial fluid) at a joint.
- CALCANEAL SPUR – abnormal sharp projection on the heel bone causing extreme pain when standing and walking.
- CALLOUS – hard and thickened skin commonly found on the soles of the feet, commonly caused by poor posture resulting from uneven distribution of body weight. May also occur on the hands due to constant pressure or friction.
- CARPAL TUNNEL SYNDROME – a condition affecting the nerves from the wrist to the hand causing pain and loss of use.
- CHILBLAINS – sore purple swellings that affect the fingers, toes and ears as a result of exposure to the cold. They may also be caused by poor circulation to the area.
- CLAW FOOT (pes cavus) – excessive arching of the foot that is usually present at birth. The foot has a high arch and clawed toes that result in a calloused sole and pain in the instep.
- CLUB FOOT – abnormality of the joints of the feet, often due to the baby lying in an abnormal position in the womb. May also be associated with cerebral palsy.
- CORN – thickening of skin on the bony points of toes and feet consisting of a central core surrounded by layers of skin. Caused by friction and pressure.
- DEAFNESS – may be congenital, temporary or associated with ageing.
- DIABETES – underproduction of insulin in the pancreas. Blood vessels to the feet may become blocked resulting in cold, painful and ulcerated feet. Sensory nerves in the hands and feet may also be affected resulting in pins and needles or numbness.
- DUPUYTREN'S CONTRACTURE – a fixed bending forward of the fingers due to the shortening and thickening of fibrous tissue in the palm.
- EARWAX – compacted earwax can cause blockage of the outer ear canal.
- EGGSHELL NAILS – very thin nails resulting from defective circulation.
- ECZEMA – a skin condition also known as DERMATITIS. There are five different types, all of which have several symptoms including redness, swelling, itchiness and blisters. A common site for eczema is the hands.
- FLAT FEET (pes planus) – natural arching of the feet develops during childhood. Lack of development results in foot strain and pain in adulthood.
- FOOT STRAIN – a straining of ligaments caused by excessive walking and/or unaccustomed foot wear.
- FURROWS – ridges in the nails that may run transversely (Beau's lines) and are associated with temporary problems

with the production of new cells, or longitudinally which are usually associated with age.

- GANGLION – a harmless swelling that often occurs at a tendon near a joint. Commonly found on the back of the wrist. Other sites include the palm of the hand, the fingers and the heel of the foot or ankle.

- GANGRENE – a lack of blood supply will cause the extremities of the body, e.g. the fingers or toes, to decay and die. Gangrene may occur as a result of diabetes, frostbite, bed sores etc.

- GOUT – a disorder affecting the chemical processes of the body. Symptoms include severe pain, swelling and redness within a joint. The joint of the big toes is most commonly affected but ankles and wrists are also common sites. In cases of chronic gout, hard lumps may develop on the ears, hands and feet.

- HAMMER TOE (pes malleus valgus) – deformity of the toes resulting in bent toes.

- HANGNAIL (agnail) – the skin around the nail becomes loose and ragged.

- HEEL FISSURES – thickened skin at the heel that forms into dry cracks.

- HIGH ARCHES (pes cavus) – feet with abnormally high arches resulting in claw foot.

- HYPERHIDROSIS – excessive sweating affecting areas such as the hands and feet. May be congenital or hormonal.

- INGROWN NAIL (onychocrytosis) – corners of the nail grow inwards piercing the surrounding skin resulting in inflammation. Usually affects the big toe.

- KERATOSIS – hard, dry, scaly, flat brown growths which often develop on the back of the hands as a result of prolonged exposure to sunshine.

- KOILONYCHIA – spoon shaped nails commonly associated with a deficiency in iron.

- LABYRINTHITIS – an inflammation of the inner ear (which is responsible for maintaining balance) resulting in dizziness and nausea.

- LEUCONYCHIA – white spots on the nail caused by a superficial knock.

- MALLET FINGER – a finger that cannot be straightened due to damage to the tendon.

- MASTOIDITIS – inflammation of the mastoid bone situated behind the ear lobe. Usually associated with a perforated eardrum.

- MENIERE'S DISEASE – a swelling of the balance mechanism of the body in the inner ear resulting in dizziness, vomiting and deafness. Only affects adults.

- MOTION SICKNESS – nausea caused by the motion associated with travelling in cars, boats and planes etc. The motion upsets the balance between what the eyes see and the inner ear feels.

Angel advice

If you feel that by working over the area you will make a condition worse it is contra indicated to treatment. Choose an alternative site.

- METATARSALGIA – the feet are flattened at the front and the toes spread out resulting in pain across the ball of the foot. Causes include bearing excessive weight due to overweight and tight fitting shoes.
- NOISE INJURY – the effects of loud noise can damage the cells of the hearing organ within the inner ear resulting in the sensation of having cotton wool in the ears, ringing in the ears and temporary or permanent deafness.
- ONYCHATROPHIA – thinning of the nail.
- ONYCHAUXIS – thickening of the nail.
- ONYCHIA – inflammation of the skin under the nail, often resulting in the loss of the nail.
- ONYCHOGRYPHOSIS – thickening and curving of the nail, causing it to become claw-like.
- ONYCHOLYSIS – separation of the nail from the underlying skin.
- ONYCHOMADESIS – complete loss of the nail.
- ONYCHOMALCIA – softening of the nail.
- ONYCHOMYCOSIS – fungal disease resulting in white, thickened nails that crumble easily.
- ONYCHOPHAGY – bitten nails.
- ONYCHOPTOSIS – shedding of the nail. May be associated with loss of hair.
- ONYCHORRHEXIS – longitudinal splitting of the nail associated with dry, brittle nails and ageing.
- ONYCHOSCHIZIA – flaking nails.
- ONYCHOTILLOMANIA – neurotic picking of the nails.
- OSTEOARTHRITIS – gradual wearing away of cartilage at a joint causing pain, swelling and deformity. Commonly affects the fingers.
- OSTEOPOROSIS – weakening of the bones which may be caused by changing levels of the hormones oestrogen and progesterone.
- OTITIS EXTERNA – infection of the outer ear canal often referred to as 'swimmer's ear' resulting in localised pain and discharge.
- OTITIS MEDIA – inflammation of the middle ear. It may be acute, which is associated with the common cold and results in earache, **chronic-secretory** also known as GLUE EAR in which the ear becomes blocked and **chronic-suppurative** which gradually damages the middle ear and ear drum.
- OTOSCLEROSIS – thickening of the bone through which sound is transmitted from the middle ear to the inner ear resulting in dizziness, ringing and deafness.
- PARONYCHIA – bacterial or fungal infection affecting the skin at the side of the nail.
- PARKINSON'S DISEASE – a condition in which muscular stiffness and tremors develop as parts of the brain degenerate leading to a deficiency of dopamine which aids the transmission of nerve impulses.

- PERFORATED EARDRUM – a hole in the eardrum caused by injury or infection.
- PIGEON TOES – turning in of toes.
- PLANTAR FASCIITIS – inflammation of the muscles in the sole of the foot resulting in acute pain in the heel when standing or walking.
- PTERYGIUM – overgrown cuticles that adhere to the nail.
- RAYNAUD'S SYNDROME – numbness and discolouration of the hands, fingers and feet affecting people who are unduly sensitive to the cold. May be associated with circulatory disorders and/or smoking.
- REPETITIVE STRAIN INJURY (RSI) – excessive, prolonged and repetitive movements cause damage to the joints resulting in swelling, pain and injury. The wrist is commonly affected. An occupational hazard for massage therapists, keyboard users etc.
- RHEUMATISM – a general term used for pain affecting the muscles and joints.
- RHEUMATOID ARTHRITIS – progressive destruction of the joints, including those of the wrists and fingers and ankles and toes, resulting in swollen, stiff joints.
- TINNITUS – ringing, buzzing or tinkling noises in the ears that have no external source. Usually associated with other ear problems.
- VERRUCA (plantar wart) – a viral infection resulting in firm, round, rough growths embedded in the soles of the feet or the toes. Blood vessels supplying the verruca can be seen beneath the skin as dark spots.
- WARTS – five types including common, plane, plantar, filiform, and anogenital. They are all caused by viruses and are contagious. Common warts are rough, skin-coloured and are generally found on the hands. Plantar warts are found on the feet (see verruca).
- WHITLOW – an infection of the soft pad of the fingers or thumb resulting in severe pain. Often confused with paronychia.

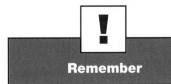

Remember

An understanding of these conditions will enable you to determine whether or not the part is indicated for treatment. If in doubt seek medical advice first e.g. a chiropodist may provide advice on foot conditions etc.

Knowledge review

1   Name the nine main systems that make up a human being.

2   Name the bones that make up the feet, ankles and toes.

3   What are the names given to the three arches of the feet?

4   Name the bones that make up the hands, wrists and fingers.

5   Name the three main sections that make up the ear.

6   What is the term given to the earflap?

7   Name the tube that links the ear with the nasopharynx.

8   What do the terms anterior, dorsal, palmar and helix mean?

9   What is the definition of contraindication?

10 What action could you take if a contraindication was present on the feet?

Practical skills

Massage forms the basis of the practical skills needed for reflexology, which may be categorised as **holding**, **relaxation**, **pressure** and **breathing techniques**.

Tip

It is useful if you have a background of experience in massage prior to training in reflexology. The movements will be easier to understand and to execute as a result of this prior knowledge.

Holding

A reflexology treatment starts with a positive touch or hold involving the initial application of the hands onto the area to be treated. This is often referred to as a 'greeting' and formally introduces the practitioner's hands to the feet, hands or ears. This

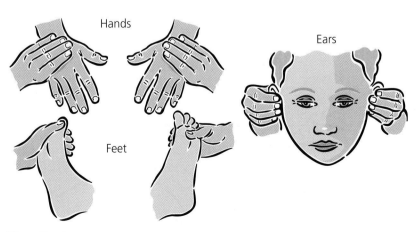

Hands

Ears

Feet

'Greeting'

technique is also used to 'close' the treatment and precipitates the final releasing of the practitioner's hands from the feet, hands or ears. The positive touch or hold may be further enhanced with the intake of a few deep breaths, visualisations and/or affirmations on the part of the client and/or practitioner relevant to either the start or the close of the reflexology treatment.

Relaxation techniques

Relaxation techniques are preparatory movements:

- Used at the start of the treatment to prepare the area *prior* to the pressure movements being performed.
- Used *after* the pressure movements have been completed in order to prepare the area for the close of the treatment.

In addition, relaxation techniques may be used at any time during a treatment to regain relaxation and in combination with breathing techniques, which are usually carried out at the start and/or the end of the treatment.

Relaxation techniques relevant to reflexology include a variety of **effleurage**, **joint manipulation**, **petrissage**, **percussion** and **vibration** movements.

Effleurage

As with all forms of massage treatment, reflexology is started, linked and completed with effleurage. Smooth, rhythmical, surface movements start the relaxation process by warming the tissue and stimulating the blood flow to the area whilst at the same time having a calming and soothing effect on the mind, inducing a sense of well-being. Movements relevant to reflexology include:

- Stroking in any direction – whole or part of the palmar surface of the hands and/or fingers/thumbs is used with

Tip

Relaxation techniques are used to warm up the area at the start of the treatment as well as to cool down the area at the end of the treatment.

Angel advice

Relaxation techniques give the practitioner the opportunity to get a feel for the feet, hands or ears and in doing so get more of a feel for their client as a whole person.

Hands   Feet   Ears

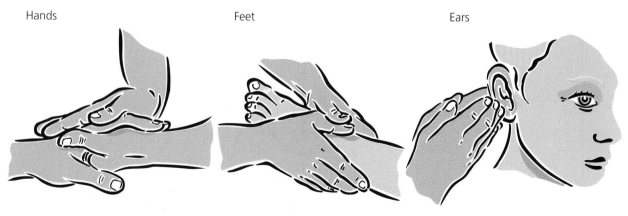

Effleurage – stroking in any direction

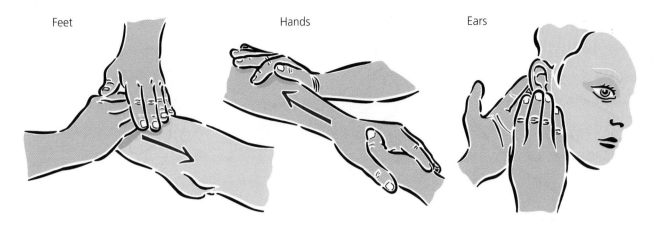

Feet   Hands   Ears

Effleurage – stroking towards the heart

equal pressure throughout the strokes. Hands are usually used alternately with one hand commencing a stroke as the other finishes and provide a means to work both sides of the body i.e. both feet, hands or ears at the same time and/or concentrate on one side or the other. Suitable for the feet, hands and ears.

● Stroking towards the heart – the whole of the palmar surface of the hands and/or fingers/thumbs is used to cover the area being treated. The pressure builds as the stroke comes to an end, helping to direct the flow of blood towards the heart and the flow of lymph towards the nearest lymph nodes. Suitable for the feet, hands and ears.

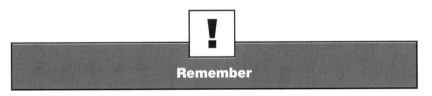

!

Remember

Direct effleurage movements towards the popliteal nodes behind the knees when treating the feet, towards the supratrochlear nodes behind the elbow when treating the hands and the auricular nodes behind the ears when treating the ears.

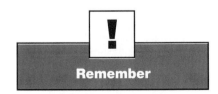

!

Remember

Synovial joints are freely moveable e.g. hinge joints of the fingers and toes.

Joint manipulations

Joint manipulations are movements which when performed assist the range of movement possible where bone meets bone. This encourages greater ease of movement in synovial joints where there may have been restriction due to over- or under-work of muscles. Movements relevant to reflexology include:

Feet   Hands   Ears

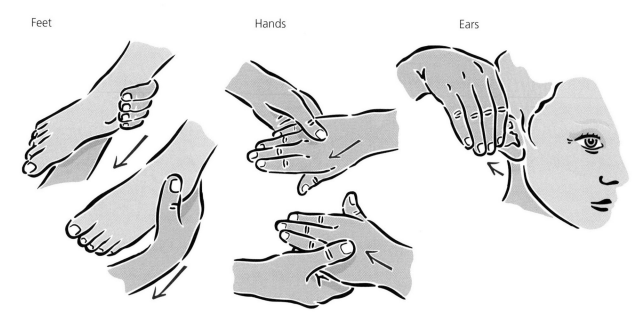

Stretch

Feet

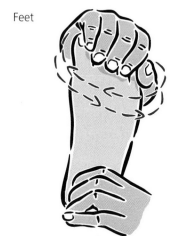

- Stretch – involving a gentle pull to the area to relieve pressure in the joints and ligaments, muscles and tendons. Suitable for the feet, hands and ears.
- Rotation – a supported movement taking a joint with rotational functions through its natural range of movements. The part is rotated first one way and then the other. Suitable for the feet – ankles and toes – and hands – wrist and fingers/thumb.
- Twist – both hands are used in a twisting motion over the area. Suitable for the feet and hands.

Hands

Feet   Hands

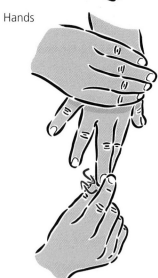

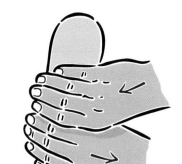

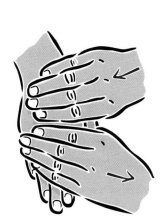

Rotation   **Twist**

Petrissage

Petrissage movements provide the means to delve deeper into the area. Firmer pressure allows deeper penetration and greater stimulation. This has the effect of 'opening' the body and thus the mind (and spirit) allowing the practitioner greater access to the body as a whole. Movements relevant to reflexology include:

- **Kneading** – the palmar surface of the hands, fingers and/or thumbs are used to perform deep pressure circles over the tissue. Suitable for feet, hands and ears.
- **Knuckling** – similar to kneading except that the top surface of the fingers is used to gently but firmly press into the tissue in a circular and/or stroking motion. Suitable for feet and hands.

Palmar kneading – hands   Palmar kneading – feet   Thumb kneading – ear

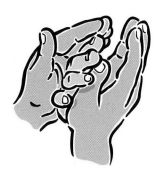
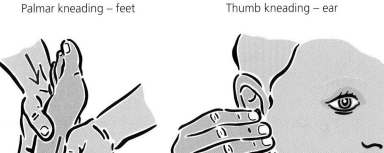

Kneading

Hands   Feet

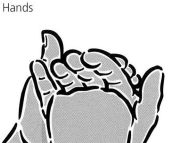
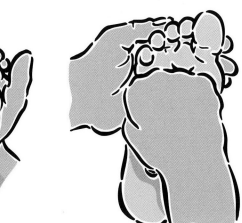

Knuckling

Tip

Because of the structure of the ear, kneading and circular friction movements may be performed with the thumb and index finger at the same time. One is used for support whilst the other performs the movement or they both work simultaneously.

● **Frictions** – the palmar surface of the fingers or thumbs are used in either a side-to-side or circular motion providing a localised deeply stimulating effect. Suitable for the feet, hands and ears.

Feet

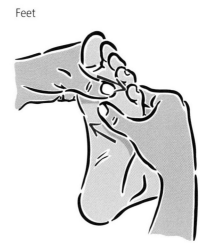

Hands

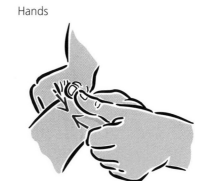

Ears

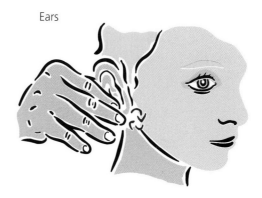

Frictions

Percussion

Percussion movements are performed quickly and briskly and have a stimulating effect on both the surface and deep tissues. Movements relevant to reflexology include:

Plucking the feet   Tapping the hands   Flicking the ears

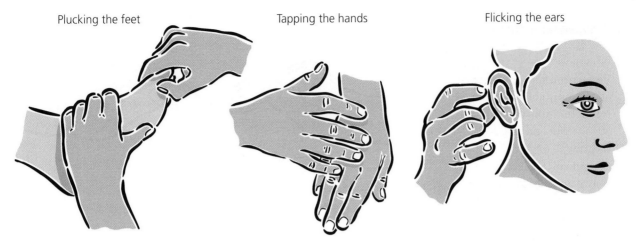

Tapotement

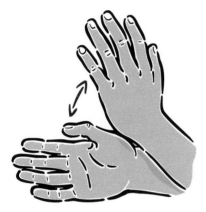

Hacking

- **Tapotement** – the tips of the fingers and thumbs are used to gently pluck, tap or flick the surface tissue. Alternate fingers/hands are used to perform quick energising movements. Suitable for the feet, hands and ears.
- **Hacking** – the lateral side of the hands is used alternately to gently strike the surface. Hands are relaxed; fingers open and elbows bent outwards with the movement coming from the wrist. Suitable for the feet and hands.
- **Pounding** – the hands are made into loose fists, which are used alternately to gently strike the surface. The lateral side of the hand (little finger side) makes contact before springing back up, making this a firm but bouncy movement. Suitable for the feet and hands.

 Angel advice

Percussion movements should be used with care, especially over bony areas. Adapt pressure to suit the area being treated, ensuring that the movements do not cause any discomfort.

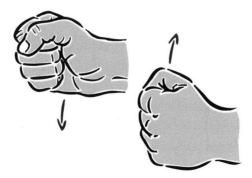

Pounding

Tip

Percussion movements are often omitted from the relaxation routine or used only at the end of the treatment to gently 'reawaken' the client, because they are noisy to perform.

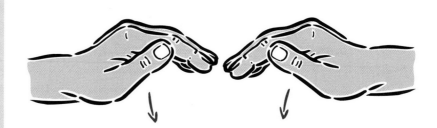

Cupping

- **Cupping** – the hands are cupped and used alternately to gently strike the surface so that the underside of the 'cup' makes contact. Suction is produced as the hands are raised, creating a stimulating effect. Suitable for the feet and hands.

Vibrations

Vibrations produce movement within the muscles helping to relieve stiffness and pain thus aiding relaxation. Movements relevant to reflexology include:

- **Shaking** – both hands are used to gently rock the area being treated. Suitable for feet and hands.

A relaxation routine will incorporate a combination of movements suited to the clients needs and will vary in the length of time it takes to perform depending on the level of relaxation required. Tense, nervous clients will need a longer relaxation time.

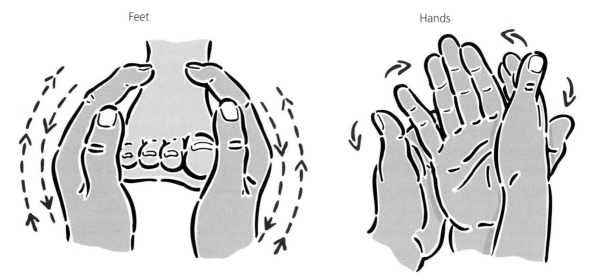

Feet

Hands

Shaking

Relaxation movements should be performed logically and intuitively. Knowledge of the movements together with their effects and benefits will ensure a suitable choice of relaxation techniques are adopted. Picking up on the needs of the client through the sense of touch, awareness of body language and adapting the movements accordingly will achieve an effective result.

Activity

Try a combination of relaxation movements on a loved one. Get them to tell you how it feels – take note of their comments and adapt your movements accordingly. Try the relaxation techniques with and without the use of a massage medium, observing the differences.

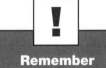

Remember

Eunice Ingham discovered that using compression movements with her fingers and thumbs proved to be the most effective form of treatment.

Tip

Stressed areas on the feet, hands and ears highlight stresses in the corresponding body parts, zones, meridians and/or chakras.

Pressure techniques

Pressure techniques incorporate alternating light and firm pressing and releasing movements on specific areas of the feet, hands and ears.

The use of these pressure/compression movements facilitates the detection of stressed areas on the feet, hands and ears and has the potential to bring about the following effects:

● Stimulate blood flow to and from the area, increasing cellular function.
● Stimulate nerve responses to and from the central nervous system.
● Stimulate energy flow within the zones, meridians and chakras.
● Free congestion and blocked energy.
● Aid relaxation and well-being.

More precision is needed when performing pressure techniques and it is for this reason that the thumb and finger pads are used (the knuckle may also be used for additional pressure if needed). Both hands are used, with one hand acting as the *working* hand and the

Angel advice

Stressed areas on the feet, hands and ears may feel hard, lumpy, granular, puffy etc. to the practitioner and scratchy, tight, painful, sharp etc. to the client.

other as the *supporting* hand when necessary. In addition, when the thumb or fingers of the working hand are performing the movement the rest of the hand acts as *leverage*, providing an anchor point. This helps to ensure greater accuracy and enables the pressure of the movement to be varied with ease.

Angel advice

Pressure techniques give the practitioner the opportunity to get an insight into the feet, hands and ears and in doing so gain a greater insight into the person as a whole.

Tip

As you place your hand on a table see how the thumb naturally lays to one side. This is the natural position for thumb walking.

Movements include **thumb walking**, **finger walking**, **thumb or finger slide**, **pivot-on-a-point**, **hook-in-back-up**, **rocking**, **thumb and finger press** and **whole hand, thumb or finger hold**.

- Thumb walking – with the thumb bent at the first joint small movements that mimic a caterpillar walking are made. The tip and pad of the thumb makes contact with the area to be treated with the pressure slightly focused on the medial side. The thumb never straightens completely but maintains a varied bend at the joint as changes in pressure take place during the 'walk'. The movements always take place in a forward motion and may run vertically, horizontally or diagonally along the area to be treated.

- Finger walking – same as thumb walking but using the fingers. The index finger is most commonly used although other fingers may also be used either singly or as a group depending on the area to be treated.

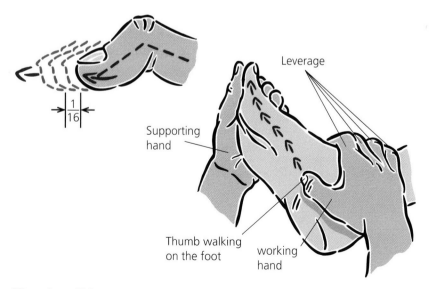

Thumb walking

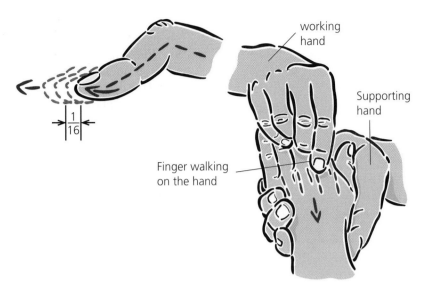

working
hand

Supporting
hand

Finger walking
on the hand

Finger walking

- Thumb or finger slide – maintaining the same position as for 'walking', the thumb or fingers gently slide back and forth over an area, moving the underlying tissue as they do so. The pressure can be easily varied and is used as a soothing movement when focusing on a specific point.

- Pivot-on-a-point – extra pressure may be applied to a specific area by focusing on the point with the thumb or finger and applying pressure in a circular motion. This is applied 'on-the-spot' as a deep movement rather than on the surface. The depth of pressure can be altered depending on the amount of leverage offered by the rest of the working hand.

- Hook-in-back-up – it is sometimes necessary to apply deeper and more specific pressure to locate a point. To do this the thumb is flexed and hooked into a point before being pulled back down. The pressure is great and should be used with care.

- Rocking – the thumb or index finger is used on the spot and gently rocked from side to side.

- Thumb and/or finger press – an on the spot press and release using the thumb and/or finger pad will help to

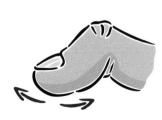

Thumb/finger slide

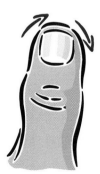

Pivot-on-a-point

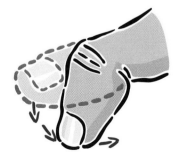

Hook-in-back-up

gently focus a specific point. Varied amounts of pressure may be used depending on the leverage.

- Whole hand, thumb and/or finger hold – a light holding technique that allows the practitioner to focus on a specific point or general area with little or no pressure. This can be used to maintain a position whilst talking to the client, to re-establish contact after a break in the treatment or to apply greater mental focus on the area.

 Activity

You can practise all of these techniques on your own feet, hands and ears adapting them accordingly. Sit on the floor supporting one foot with your corresponding leg and practice thumb walking along the zones on the sole. Try finger walking along the back of your hand from the base of the fingers to the wrist. Use thumb/finger press movements along your ears. Try a combination of other techniques as you feel areas of tension in your feet, hands and ears.

Pressure techniques should be performed slowly, rhythmically and in a relaxed manner. Think about your posture and try to relax as much as possible. Allow your senses to help you to focus on the movements so that they become natural and eventually intuitive. Never try to force the movements, instead try to open your mind and learn to go with the flow. You will soon learn to work instinctively in a way that feels right for both you and your client.

 Activity

Practise the movements using both hands so that your pressure is balanced between the left and right side of your body. Whilst practising, pay particular attention to what your support hand is doing. Extreme concentration on the working hand may lead to excessive squeezing with the support hand, which could cause discomfort. Start with relaxation movements, using a massage medium if required. Continue with pressure movements without adding any additional product. Complete with relaxation movements.

Breathing techniques

Breathing techniques form an important part of the treatment for both the practitioner and the client and may be used in two ways:

- Breathing exercises – taking time out at the start and/or end of the treatment to practise deep-breathing exercises aids relaxation and provides a positive focus for the treatment. Visualisations and affirmations may be incorporated with the breathing, concentrating on drawing in positivity with the inward breath and releasing negativity with the outward breath. This has the effect of helping to clear the mind and balance the body systems in preparation for the treatment as well as bring the body and mind back to reality at the close of the treatment.

- Pressure breathing – incorporating the application of pressure to a point on the feet, hands or ears with the inward breath to energise whilst focusing on the release of tension as the pressure releases with the outward breath. Visualisations add to the effectiveness of this technique as the practitioner and client imagine the process with their mind's eye. Affirmations can also provide access to greater release as the use of sound amplifies the therapeutic effects. Pressure breathing can be used at any time throughout the treatment and is especially beneficial when focusing on a stressed area.

As we have seen, our hands provide the best tools for the practical application of a reflexology treatment and as such should be well cared for. There should be balance between the pressure and coordination applied by both the left and the right hands despite having a dominant side i.e. being either left- or right-handed. Hand exercises that encourage the development of hand and eye coordination as well as strength building are a beneficial way of developing these vital tools.

In addition, the hands are common sites for the effects of stress as there is a tendency to hold on to tension both physically and emotionally as a person responds to the strains of everyday living. Stress and tension may build up in the hands in either or both of the following ways:

Tip

Good coordination of both hands demonstrates excellent links between the left and right hemispheres of the brain.

Feet   Hands   Ears

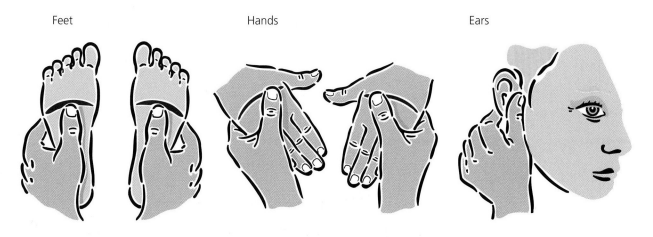

Pressure breathing

- As part of the appendicular skeleton forming an extension of the main body, the hands take on board the tension that builds up in the back, shoulders and arms.
- Tension tends to build up in the hands as a result of the many activities they are called upon to perform during the course of day.

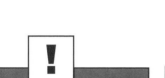

Remember

The thumb and fingers need to be sensitive to touch in order to pick up on any imbalance. It is impossible to achieve this if the hands are poorly cared for. Your hands really are the tools of your trade!

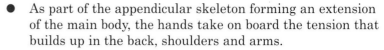

Activity

After a long and stressful day, feel the tension that has built up in your own hands. Notice the tightness and stiffness in the hands as the flexor and extensor muscles have become fatigued. You may experience a reduction in strength and a loss of coordination as a result. Carry out some of the relaxation techniques on yourself – or better still, get someone else to do them for you!

Angel advice

Nails should be short, evenly filed and free of enamel. Hands should be kept moisturised and exercised.

Stress relieving exercises are vital if the hands are to be at their best to perform the practical skills associated with giving a reflexology treatment. The condition of the skin and nails are also a consideration in the care and presentation of the hands. Reddened dry hands and uneven, split nails for example give a visual impression of lack of care – if a practitioner of reflexology cannot take care of themselves how can a client be expected to have confidence in their skills in caring for them! In addition, rough hands and ragged nails prevent a smooth, flowing treatment from taking place and so general care and consideration of the hands should become a daily task for the reflexology practitioner.

Knowledge review

1 Which movements are used as a greeting at the start of the treatment?

2 Give five different types of relaxation movements that may be used in reflexology.

3 Give four benefits of relaxation movements.

4 Give three reasons for the use of pressure techniques during a reflexology treatment.

5 Which part of the hands performs the pressure techniques?

6 Give five different pressure techniques.

7 Why is it important to perform pressure techniques slowly?

8 Give two reasons why breathing techniques can be included within a reflexology treatment.

9 Give two ways in which stress builds up in the hands.

10 Give three ways in which care can be taken to ensure the hands are in a suitable condition to give reflexology treatments.

Psychological skills

Psychological skills are those that are associated with the mind –
some we can quantify, others are not so easily described. The
quantifiable skills are those generally associated with the left
hemisphere of the brain and logical thought e.g. we can logically
assume that if someone says that they are happy then they are.
However the activity in the right hemisphere of the brain may lead
us to a different conclusion as we intuitively pick up on the fact
that the same person seems unhappy. We may find it easier to
trust the logical thought than the intuitive one, because we have
more proof and find it more difficult to go with our gut reaction
because we are afraid of being wrong. Experience of life enables us
to make these decisions more easily and as such life skills form an
important part of the client/practitioner relationship. However, we
can also learn to make use of our inborn skills more effectively and
to develop new ones that may be used to enhance the reflexology
treatment.

Tip

A balance between logical and intuitive thought is the aim of
the reflexology practitioner.

Remember that reflexology is a two-way treatment requiring the
involvement of both the client and the practitioner. This
client/practitioner relationship commonly goes through three main
phases and levels of dependency.

- Phase one – the client identifies that they have a problem
  and seeks treatment. The client is effectively saying 'help
  me' and the emphasis is placed on the skills of the
  practitioner. The client is often totally dependent on the
  practitioner in terms of their well-being e.g. when they
  should have a treatment, how often etc.

Tip

Affirmations and
visualisations are also
classed as mind skills –
mental processes which
people can be trained in
and/or train themselves
which help to focus the
mind on the positive.

Angel advice

CPD (continued
professional development)
is a result of increased self-
awareness and should form
an integral part of every
practitioner's working life.

Tip

Communication is a means
of conveying a message and
counselling conveys a
message in a helpful
manner.

- Phase two – if the practitioner's skills are effective then they will encourage the client to work with them to achieve a greater sense of awareness in their own ability to help themselves. The emphasis shifts as dependency on the practitioner lessens and the treatment becomes more client-centred.

- Phase three – the aim of the practitioner should be to build on this awareness until the client is able to ascertain what they need and when in terms of their own treatment. The client then becomes independent and more in control of their own well-being.

To become effective as a practitioner of reflexology and practice a truly holistic approach we should aim to develop certain mind skills. Awareness forms the basis of such skills, including self-awareness and client-awareness.

Self-awareness

Self-awareness forms the starting point of the treatment. It highlights our strengths and weaknesses and determines our limitations. By identifying these factors we can aim to work on improving our effectiveness through further training as well as through experiential learning without ever taking on anything that is beyond our capabilities or limitations.

Client-awareness

Client-awareness forms the development of the treatment. It highlights the client's holistic needs, enabling the practitioner to adapt their skills accordingly. Having such awareness enables the practitioner to potentially take the client through the physical, emotional and spiritual levels of the treatment. This ensures that the treatment remains effective for the client and challenging for the practitioner.

The means of achieving both self- and client-awareness is through the developing use of **communication** and **counselling** skills.

Communication skills

Communication is a two-way process that incorporates the use of our whole being to receive and convey messages between other beings.

Communication skills incorporate the ability to:

- Detect and receive messages through our sensory organs i.e. skin, nose, eyes, ears and tongue.

- Interpret the messages through our central nervous system i.e. brain and spinal cord.

- Relay messages back through our whole body.

Communication is therefore physical, psychological as well as spiritual and may be classified as being **verbal** and **non-verbal**.

Verbal communication

We use the art of speaking to communicate with the world around us through verbal and vocal messages. Verbal messages are what is said with words; vocal messages include those messages sent through the voice by the use of:

- Sound – the volume, pitch and tone of the voice will relay a mixture of messages e.g. when communicating anger we tend to raise the volume of the voice.
- Speed – the rate at which one speaks relays the feelings associated with the message being communicated e.g. an overworked, stressed person tends to speak quickly.
- Articulation – the use of words helps to ensure effective communication of a specific message.
- Emphasis – the force with which the words are being expressed helps to relay the importance of the message.

Non-verbal communication

We use our whole body to communicate with the world around through **bodily**, **tactile** and **thought messages**.

Bodily messages

Bodily messages form the basis of face-to-face communication and include:

- Facial expressions – the easiest of all bodily messages to control, but they will portray a reaction to what is being said and heard e.g. a smile makes a greeting so much more welcoming.
- Eye contact – whether or not we look at a person and how long for whilst speaking or listening to them determines the levels of sincerity and interest in what is being said or heard e.g. eye contact is usually broken if someone is attempting to lie.
- Eye movements – used to convey interest, to gain feedback, to synchronise speech and to show attraction. Some eye movements are quite uncontrollable yet send out very strong messages e.g. when we see something that attracts us the pupils dilate.
- Posture – the way a person stands or sits will help to portray the true message they are trying to communicate e.g. if a person sits facing another person it sends out a message of interest; if they sit with their legs facing in another direction it clearly demonstrates their lack of interest.

Fascinating Fact

We often refer to a person who uses lots of gestures as someone who 'talks with their hands'.

Fascinating Fact

Different cultures determine the acceptance of differing levels of proximity between people.

Fascinating Fact

School teachers are discouraged from hugging school children in case their action is misinterpreted, despite the fact that sometimes a hug is more important than a word.

Fascinating Fact

Research in Norway has shown that teenagers prefer to communicate through text messages rather than face-to-face!

- Gestures – parts of the body are used to communicate strong messages such as information and emotion and/or to express self-image e.g. an extrovert person often expresses themselves with energetic gestures whilst a shy person is more restricted in their use of gestures.

- Appearance – physical grooming and choice of clothes project very strong messages associated with image.

- Proximity – the distance we keep from one another helps to communicate the type of relationship message e.g. intimate (from half a metre to actual touching), personal (from half to 1.25 metres), social (from 1.25 to 4 metres) and public (from 4 to 8 metres or more).

 Activity

Think about the messages sent out when a person is wearing the uniform associated with their work compared to those that are associated with leisure clothes.

Tactile messages

Tactile messages are those conveyed through touch and are thought to be amongst the earliest form of communication. Touch is often avoided as a means of communication because it may be open to misinterpretation. Consideration must be paid to:

- Permission – touch is a two-way method of communication that requires agreement.
- Pressure – touch involves varying depths of pressure that should meet the agreed needs.

Thought messages

Thought messages form the basis of *non* face-to-face communication and include:

- Written communication – the written word is a powerful means of communication as is the way in which it has been written e.g. the study of personality types through handwriting styles is a popular way of interpreting hidden messages.

- Extra-sensory communication – this refers to those methods of communication that we have no logical explanation for e.g. when the telephone rings and the person at the other end is the person we have just been thinking of.

Communication skills are never used in isolation but in combination with a variety of other related and non-related skills, often making the resulting messages confusing. As a result mixed messages are often sent out, which contributes to the difficulty in interpreting their true meaning. In addition to this there may also be barriers to communication including:

- Personality – differences in people's personalities and their resulting behaviour can cause personality clashes, which has the potential to hinder communication.
- Emotions – strong emotions such as anger and fear prevent almost everything else from being communicated.
- Language – the use of jargon and unfamiliar words put pressure on communication, shifting the power to the one with the knowledge of the words whilst the other person feels vulnerable and unable to respond.
- Stereotyping – assuming that everyone fits into a 'type' and not picking up on individualism.
- Perception – seeing things from only one point of view depending on our culture, sex, status, education etc. hinders effective communication.

A balanced use of all communication skills helps to break down these barriers and is an important factor in the treatment of clients through reflexology.

 Activity

Analyse your own communication skills by keeping a diary. Note the times you used your skills effectively compared to the times when your skills did not work so well. Think about the intent of your actions compared with the reactions – did they match.

Counselling skills

The use of counselling skills is also a two-way process and should not be confused with counselling by a qualified counsellor.

Counselling may be viewed as consisting of an approach, skills and goals within a set of boundaries governed by a strict code of ethics as laid down by the British Association of Counsellors (BAC):

- Counselling approach – a way of understanding and caring.
- Counselling skills – behaving in an understanding and caring way.
- Counselling goals – use of understanding and caring to achieve set aims.

A trained counsellor will use all three factors during a counselling session which will be conducted formally within set boundaries including:

- The session is set for an agreed period of time e.g. one hour.
- The client knows that it is a counselling session.
- There is an agreed agenda.

Many other professionals make use of counselling skills but have a different approach, set of goals and boundaries. Teachers, doctors and nurses are examples of professionals who use counselling skills to enhance their existing skills.

Activity

Each of us has our own inbuilt way of counselling that is partly instinctive and partly drawn from our own unique set of experiences. Think about the way in which you use your own skills and watch how others use theirs. Think about the ways in which people respond to your ways and how you respond to others. There are many lessons that may be learned in this way.

Practitioners of all complementary therapies including reflexology are also encouraged to make use of counselling skills in order to achieve greater levels of self- and client-awareness. The approach to reflexology treatment is holistic, the skills are theoretical, practical and psychological and adapted to meet the needs of the client, the goal is to improve well-being and the boundaries include the industry codes of practice, limits of individual expertise and treatment time:

- Industry codes of practice – a set guide to health, safety and welfare.

Activity

Get a copy of an industry code of practice and check the boundaries. You can obtain this from your training provider, awarding body or reflexology association.

- Limits of individual expertise – referral of clients to other professionals if unable to treat them.

Activity

We may refer a client with a contraindication to their GP. Make a list of other situations that may involve you referring a client to another professional.

Activity

Make a list of the reasons why it is important to place a realistic time limit on treatment.

Tip

Many clients enter reflexology treatment with curiosity and/or scepticism. A well-trained and intuitive practitioner will do much to fuel their client's curiosity and dispel their scepticism with clear explanations and effective treatments.

- Treatment time – initial treatment is approximately one and-a-quarter hours, subsequent treatments are 45–60 minutes.

The use of counselling skills can be used to enhance the reflexology treatment both for the practitioner and the client and may be applied in four stages:

- Stage one *exploring* – forming a relationship with the client through consultation and treatment.
- Stage two *understanding* – identifying a pattern of imbalance through further treatments.
- Stage three *building* – developing awareness of how positive changes could be made.
- Stage four *action* – initiating changes.

All four stages rely on specific values including **integrity** and **respect** on the part of the client and the practitioner:

- Integrity – both the practitioner and client should enter the treatment with honesty if it is to be successful.
- Respect – mutual respect should exist between the practitioner and the client as well as for the treatment itself.

Stage one

The psychological skills associated with **listening**, **empathy**, **openness** and **acceptance** are required of the practitioner:

Listening – by using sensory skills associated with our ears to hear the sounds and the interpretation skills associated with our brain to listen to the meaning we are engaging in active listening. It is also important to hear and to listen to the contributory factors that underline the sounds including:

- The tone of voice – does the tone match the use of the words? This will enable you to make a better interpretation.
- The level of breathing – is the breathing shallow, normal, deep? This will help you to pick up on the stress levels associated with what the client is saying.
- The accompanying facial and body expressions – do the expressions match the use of the words? This will help to give meaning to the words being spoken.
- The silences – it is important to pick up on what is being left unsaid. Silences provide meaningful gaps in the conversation.
- The content – it is important to link what is being said to every other factor of what you hear so that a client feels that they have been heard.

Empathy – we need to try to get a view of what the client is feeling from their perspective rather than our own. To do this we need to:

- Listen sensitively – encourage the client to talk openly by showing an interest.
- Attempt to make sense of what you hear – confirm with the client what it is you are hearing.
- Understand the person in their own terms – try to put yourself in the client's position and see things from their point of view.
- Check to see if you have listened and heard correctly – by putting into your own words your interpretation of the meaning of their words.

Openness – whilst we do not have to agree with everyone's values and opinions, we need to be open to the fact that these differ from person to person and approach each new client and situation with an open heart and mind. In doing so we need to employ the following:

- Our real self – not trying to be someone or something that we are not.
- Genuine care – really wanting to help.
- Lack of front or façade – not giving the wrong outward appearance.
- Sincerity – being truthful and tactful.

As a result of openness on the part of the practitioner, clients will feel in a better position to be open themselves.

Acceptance – in order for a client to open up they need to feel safe and secure. The client needs to feel that the practitioner offers them a psychological environment that is:

- Non-judgemental – the client needs to feel that you will not criticise or undermine their intelligence.
- Warm – your body language should reflect a welcoming manner.
- Comfortable – a client should feel as though they can say whatever it is they have to without fear of embarrassment etc.
- Supportive – a client may need encouragement e.g. in terms of finding the right words to express their meaning without putting words into their mouth.
- Positive – a means of combating the negative and of finding good from bad.
- Exclusive – a client needs to feel that their time with you is for them and them alone.
- Confidential – a client needs to know that anything they say is kept between the confines of the treatment and not discussed with any one else without their permission.

Angel advice

It is important that the client has this time to get to know the practitioner in a suitable environment if the treatment is to progress successfully. It is therefore important not to rush and to allow the client to control the speed at which the relationship develops.

Stage two

Once a relationship has been formed and the client is prepared to take the treatment a stage further, strategies can be employed to

Tip

This method is often referred to as 'reflection'. The practitioner reflects or mirrors what is being said by the client to confirm understanding.

begin to get an understanding of the messages associated with the thoughts, feelings and behaviour that have emerged from the initial treatments. To accurately clarify their meaning, the use of paraphrasing can help i.e. put into your own words what you are hearing. To do this we need to:

● Be specific – avoid generalising.
● Do not debate – it is not a discussion.
● Do not push for information – accept the client's own pace.
● Do not guess – they are the expert of their own feelings not you!

These skills may be employed to act as a sorting system for incoming information, highlighting areas that it might be useful to explore. As a result of this process the practitioner is able to:

● Summarise what has been said.
● Check their understanding.
● Focus on a particular aspect for further treatment.

Stage three

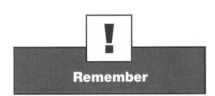

Remember

Clients will seek reflexology treatment at any stage of this development and the time associated with stages one and two helps to determine this. It is also worth remembering that clients who are not currently experiencing any of these stages of development may also seek treatments.

Increasing general awareness in this way often highlights a distortion in a person's view of themselves or their situation. This is sometimes referred to as a blind spot, and stage three helps to establish a new perspective. This facilitates a shift in focus encouraging a client to view the bigger picture.

However, a person may find themselves stuck in this distorted view and need to work through the various stages of development before being able to move on. Stages of development include:

● Shock – a period of time of realisation that something traumatic is happening or has happened.
● Denial – a period of time whereby a person cannot accept what has happened – wanting to turn back the clock.
● Depression – a period of time when a person feels unable to move on because they feel there is nothing to move on to.
● Acceptance – a period of time when a person is able to come to terms with the fact that something has happened and that life goes on.

Different people and situations determine the amount of time spent at each stage and the severity of each stage. The skills associated with stage three may be classified as *challenging*.

Challenging needs to be done carefully and tactfully and may be used to confront certain situations, for example:

● The client who does not stop talking throughout the treatment – may be challenged as to the real reason for treatment. They may be hiding the truth within the barrage of words and need help in disengaging what they mean from what they are saying rather than saying what they think they mean.

 Activity

We often refer to someone who talks incessantly as having 'verbal diarrhoea'. Think about the times this has happened to you and the associated feelings it evokes.

- The client who punctuates their sentences with lots of silences – may be challenged to ascertain the meaning of what is being left unsaid. Hidden meaning often accompanies silence and the client may need help allowing this to emerge.

 Activity

We often talk about being on the same wavelength as someone. Think about the times you have experienced this with another person and the ease with which you are able to interact with one another.

- The client who uses avoidance tactics to ignore the problem – may be gently challenged to bring the focus back to the real issue.

 Angel advice

Trust your instincts – learn to pick up on how a situation feels and adapt accordingly. If it feels right – be brave enough to go with it and if it feels wrong be strong enough to admit it and change your method or refer to someone who has the knowledge and skill to help to make it right.

 Activity

In certain situations we may experience a time when we seem to connect with another person. Think about the way this may help to guide a person to accept the challenge as part of their development.

As a practitioner of reflexology it is important to be aware of when you are able to help the personal development of your client and when you need to refer the client to a specialist because the level of your expertise does not match the level of their development. In referring the client to a specialist counsellor, e.g. for marriage guidance etc., you may continue to work with the client in order to enhance their development generally.

Stage four

Once a person has reached the stage of acceptance of their situation they are in a position to move on. However, it is not always clear in which direction they should move and so a period of time looking at the available options for change forms the basis of stage four. The development of a plan may be established that helps to action the proposed changes in the form of:

- A wish – long-term
- An aim – medium-term
- A goal – short-term.

An example might be a person's long-term **wish** to be happy. Acceptance that happiness can be found in the simplest of things may form the short-term goal, with the medium-term **aim** being to bring about some changes in life to ensure that it includes realistic activities that make that person happier.

Such a task is often difficult to do alone as one loses sight of the bigger picture and sees only the restrictions of one's current situation. However, by using counselling skills a reflexology practitioner can effectively help such a client to move on by encouraging a different viewpoint. Creative thinking provides the basis for change in the form of:

- Prompting – suggesting people, places, organisations, skills, examples etc. that may help to focus the mind on achieving rather than giving up.
- Brainstorming – encouraging bizarre and wild thoughts that at first seem totally unachievable; but the mere fact that they have been voiced makes their reality more achievable.
- Divergent thought – trying to think of several ways in which to achieve change, highlighting that there is usually more than one option. Choice provides an element of control and empowerment.

The use of communication and counselling skills incorporates a great deal of energy on the part of the client and practitioner.

Tip

It is important to appreciate that whilst creative thinking is the skill, reality is the tool and that any proposed change should be achievable. Change then becomes positive and forms a stepping-stone from a short-term goal to a medium-term aim to a long-term wish.

Activity

Think about the way you feel when you have communicated great anger or sadness as well as how you feel when someone has offloaded their anger or sadness onto you.

As a result both parties may potentially feel drained and depleted of energy, both physically and psychologically.

Strong emotions often accompany such development and as a result a form of 'healing crisis' may occur. This may involve a period of time when a person may feel worse before feeling better. A good example of this is to have a good cry. The act of crying seems a negative activity and one associated with physical and/or psychological pain, but the resulting relief experienced after crying has a far-reaching effect that is both positive and healing.

Because of this it is necessary for client and practitioner to observe certain safety measures including:

Angel advice

As a practitioner of reflexology you should ensure that you also receive the treatment on a regular basis.

- Control – the client must be given complete control over what they say and do during the treatment without ever feeling pressurised in any way. The practitioner should never treat a client beyond the scope of their knowledge and skill, referring a client when necessary.

- Protection – the client must always be protected in terms of their health, safety and welfare as well as confidentiality and privacy. They should also be given the benefit of adequate time for treatment and recovery in order to protect against unnecessary adverse reactions. The practitioner should also be protected in terms of health, safety and welfare by following the necessary legislation. It is also important that the practitioner ensures coping strategies are in place to counteract the strain of working with stressed clients.

Angel advice

We may use visualisations and/or affirmations to protect us e.g. some people may like to visualise a protective bubble or light surrounding them, others may prefer to use their inner voice to affirm their protection.

Remember

If you do not use your skills – you will lose them.

The use of theoretical, practical and psychological skills forms the basic requisites for performing the reflexology treatment. It is important to appreciate that whilst these skills may be taught and learnt the real acquisition of knowledge is in using them.

Knowledge review

1 Name the two main methods of communication.

2 Give three barriers to effective communication.

3 What is the difference between communication and counselling skills?

4 Which organisation sets the strict code of ethics that govern counsellors?

5 What are the boundaries surrounding the use of counselling skills by a reflexology practitioner?

6 What is the difference between hearing and listening?

7 What are the four common stages of development?

8 Describe a way in which one might use challenging techniques to aid personal development.

9 What are the differences between a wish, aim and goal in terms of time?

10 Why might a client and/or practitioner feel drained as a result of treatment?

Part 3

The consultation

Learning objectives

After reading this part you should be able to:

- **Recognise the need for a consultation to take place.**

- **Identify the processes involved in conducting a consultation.**

- **Understand the importance of conducting a professional consultation.**

- **Be aware of the links between an effective consultation and an effective treatment.**

- **Begin to appreciate the skills required to undertake a consultation.**

The consultation is conducted in three main stages. The first stage is predominantly paper based, whereby the practitioner takes a client case history; the second involves a practical examination of the area to be treated. The third stage is associated with treatment outcomes and recommendations for further treatment and homecare.

Consultation – stage one

8

The **consultation** process begins from the moment a client makes an initial enquiry about the reflexology treatment and is a continuous and progressive process that forms the basis of every subsequent treatment, drawing on all of the skills discussed in Part 2.

The primary aim of the consultation is to ensure that the proposed treatment is suitable for the client's needs; as a result it is a very personal and potentially invasive and intrusive process. The secondary aims should therefore be to ensure that the consultation is conducted in a sensitive and thoughtful manner, paying particular attention to the client's reasons for treatment and expectations of the treatment. These reasons and expectations are often varied and range from being very realistic in nature i.e. 'I understand that reflexology can help with stress relief' to being totally unrealistic i.e. 'I want reflexology to cure my illness now!'

In order to ascertain whether or not a client is suitable for a reflexology treatment a number of checks need to undertaken with the client's consent including:

- *Personal check:* including full name, address and telephone number. This information enables a practitioner to contact their client in the event of having to cancel or rearrange an appointment. It is also useful to get other personal information with the client's permission such as date of birth, doctor's details, profession, marital status, whether or not they have children, height and weight, their reasons for seeking treatment and their general expectations. This information provides an initial insight that goes beyond first impressions, helping to paint a picture of the client, their personal situation and their needs.

- *Medical health:* including details of pregnancy, medication, surgical operations and any other complaints that currently require medical attention or have done in the past – illnesses, allergies, hereditary diseases etc. This information helps to determine the area for treatment e.g.

Tip

Factors relating to contraindications include whether or not the client needs to seek medical approval prior to treatment in the case of a condition that may prevent treatment as well as provide the practitioner with a set of guidelines for treatment in the event of a contraindication which may restrict treatment (Part 4 gives specific contra-indication guidelines for each body system).

treating the hands if there has been a recent operation on the feet etc. It is also useful at this stage to ask the client how they view their general state of health and to include questions relating to whether or not they are or have been a smoker. This helps to lead onto the more detailed questions of the next stage of the consultation as well as provide greater access to the client's individual needs as they see them.

- *Physical health:* including questions relating to the physical well-being of the body as a whole and of the individual body systems, respiratory, digestive, reproductive etc. This information helps to highlight possible stresses with the direct and associated symptoms e.g. constipation puts stress on the body and such a condition will alert us to the digestive system because of the direct symptoms of congestion in the large intestines which will have a knock-on effect on the other parts of the system. However, other systems of the body may also be affected and associated symptoms may include skin problems, lack of energy etc. (Part 4 provides detailed explanation of the specific anatomy and physiology of each body system).

- *Emotional health:* including details of how the client relates to stress, tension, anxiety and depression. This information helps to ascertain how the client views themselves in terms of their emotional welfare and how much support they are going to need in terms of their quest for well-being. Our constipated client, for example, may find that their skin is causing them concern and as a result is feeling anxious. They may start to experience a loss of confidence and decreasing self-esteem. In addition, some people say that they are feeling depressed because things in their life are bad and they feel they can only get worse. Their negative attitude can prove to be a barrier to well-being and potentially they will need more support – possibly more than you are able to give without referring them to a specialist. Another person in the same or similar situation will express a more positive outlook, saying that things are bad now but will get better. Their potential for well-being is improved by their positive attitude and they are likely to need less support. This information also helps to highlight the links between emotional and physical well-being and the knock-on effect that one has on the other.

- *Lifestyle:* including details relating to work, leisure, diet and exercise. This information helps to ascertain the likely causes of stress-related symptoms e.g. overwork, lack of free time, poor eating habits and lack of exercise are all associated with stress. There may be additional personal or professional stresses involved contributing to a short-term problem which, if not addressed, have the potential to create medium- and even long-term physical and/or emotional problems.

The way in which the questions relating to these factors are asked is a crucial part of the consultation process, providing the key to gaining a person's trust and respect. Care should be taken to present questions that can be seen as being justifiable (the client needs to understand the reasons why you are asking such questions) and that are:

- Open – questions that encourage the client to answer with a sentence rather than with a positive or a negative e.g. 'How are you feeling today?' instead of 'Are you feeling well today?'

- Follow-up – questions that help to gain more specific information e.g. 'How often do you feel this way?' and 'How do you cope?' etc.

- Unthreatening – questions that make a client feel safe so that they can be free to answer honestly e.g. 'It is amazing how little water the average person drinks on a daily basis. How much do you tend to drink?' instead of 'We should all drink at least eight glasses of water a day. Do you drink that many?'

- Jargon free – questions that avoid the use of technical terms that a client may not know the meaning of and which have the potential of making them feel uncomfortable and lacking in knowledge e.g. 'How often do you find yourself shallow breathing?' instead of 'How often are you practising apical breathing'.

- Non-judgemental – questions that do not offer an opinion or criticism e.g. 'How would you describe your smoking habit?' instead of 'Don't you think that smoking 30 cigarettes a day is a bit excessive?'

- Clarifying – questions that allow you to check details e.g. to clarify a type of medication you may not have heard of and do not know what it is for. To clarify the spelling of a word you are unfamiliar with.

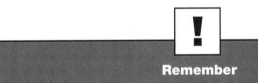

Remember

A reflexology practitioner is not a doctor and as such is not expected to know every medical detail, so do not be afraid to ask.

Remember

Your tone of voice will contribute to the way in which the questions are interpreted.

- Linking – questions that help you to link systems and symptoms e.g. 'You have said that you have problems with your digestive system in terms of indigestion and a bloated feeling after eating lunch. Do you tend to eat your lunch "on the run"?' etc.

The first stage of the consultation process may be divided into five distinct phases – **preparation, introduction, case history, explanation** and **confirmation**:

REFLEXOLOGY
CONSULTATION FORM – STAGE ONE

Name .... Date ....

Address .... Tel. No work ....

.... Tel. No home ....

....Tel. No mobile ....

Date of birth ....

Doctors' details ....

Marital status .... Children .... ages ....

Height .... Weight ....

Reason for treatment ....

Expectation of treatment ....

Medical health

● Pregnancy ....

● Medication ....

● Operations and dates ....

● Major illnesses and dates ....

● Allergies ....

● Hereditary illness ....

● Smoker .... Frequency .... Amount ....

● Client's view of general state of health ....

Physical health – condition of and/or problems associated with:

Integumentary system

● Skin ....

● Hair ....

● Nails ....

Muscular/Skeletal system

● Bones .... Muscles ....

● Neck .... Back ....

● Shoulders .... Hips ....

● Knees .... Elbows ....

● Ankles .... Wrist ....

Respiratory system

● Hay fever .... Ashma ....

● How many times a year do you get a cold? ....

Which part(s) does it affect –

Head .... Chest .... Throat .... Sinuses .... Ears .... Eyes .... Nose ....

REFLEXOLOGY
CONSULTATION FORM – STAGE ONE *(continued)*

Circulatory systems

- Blood pressure .... Pulse rate ....
- Varicose veins .... Tired legs ....
- Fluid retention .... Cellulite ....

Digestive system

- Teeth .... Taste ....
- Eating .... Drinking ....
- Indigestion .... Bloated ....
- Constipation .... Diarrhoea ....

Urinary system

- Kidneys ....
- Bladder ....

Reproductive system

Females:

- Regular periods .... Date of last period ....
- Period now? .... Day .... Flow ....
- Contraception .... Pregnancy ....

Males:

- Prostate gland ....

Nervous system

- Headaches .... Migraine ....
- Pins and needles .... Numbness ....
- Cold hands and feet ....
- Eyesight ....

Endocrine system

- PMT ....
- Menopause .... HRT ....
- Mood swings? ....

Emotional health – rate 1–10 (1 = low, 10 = high)

- Stress levels .... details ....
- Anxiety .... details ....
- Tension .... details ....
- Depression .... details ....

REFLEXOLOGY
CONSULTATION FORM – STAGE ONE *(continued)*

Lifestyle

Work

- Profession ....
- Typical working hours ....
- Breaks? .... Frequency .... Length ....

Leisure

- Ability to relax .... Activities ....
- Hobbies .... Interests ....
- Sleep pattern .... Energy levels ....

Diet

- Preferences (vegetarian, vegan etc) ....
- How many meals per day .... Supplements ....
- Fresh fruit/veg per day .... Protein ....
- Carbohydrate .... Fats ....
- Dairy products .... Additives (salt, sugar etc.) ....
- Water per day .... Tea/coffee/cola per day ....
- Fruit juice per day .... Alcohol per day. ....
- Herbal tea per day .... Type .... Reason ....
- Details of food/fluid intake today ....
  ....
  ....

Exercise

- Type .... Frequency ....

Additional info

- Use of sunbed .... Sunscreen ....
- Posture check ....
- Anything else client would like to discuss ....
- Any questions ....
  ....
  ....

The information I have given is correct to the best of my knowledge.

I have been fully informed about contraindications.

I am happy to proceed with the treatment.

Client signature ....

Practitioner signature ....

Angel advice

When setting up a consultation/treatment area it may be useful to consider the principles of Feng Shui which can help to ensure a free flow of energy and the potential to enhance any activity within the space provided (see the A–Z of complementary therapies in Chapter 4).

Preparation

An effective treatment relies on an efficient consultation, so thought should be given to:

- *Environment* – this should be private and out of sight and earshot of other clients. It should be comfortable and inviting, safe and warm. Seats for the practitioner and client should be of equal height, facing one another at an appropriate angle and distance. This ensures eye contact at an equal level, which in turn sets the level of the relationship, which should also be equal. Avoid sitting behind a desk or table as this creates a physical and psychological barrier between the practitioner and client. Heating and lighting should be checked and it is necessary to ensure that there is adequate access and provision for disabled clients e.g. wheelchair, guide dog etc.

- *Tools and equipment* – a consultation form and pen should be ready for use together with any other resources you may want to use to supplement your consultation e.g. foot, hand or ear charts etc. It is useful to have sight of a clock in order to check the timing of the consultation. A box of tissues should be on hand (a consultation can in some cases evoke an emotional response) and antiseptic wipes should be available in the event of having to check the area to be treated.

- *Practitioner* – attention should be paid to the way in which you present yourself to the client. All aspects of your personal appearance should be considered in order to convey a professional image appropriate to your workplace. In particular care should be taken to ensure that your outfit is appropriate, hands are clean and soft, nails are enamel free and short and hair is tied back away from the face. Jewellery should be kept to a minimum for safety reasons and due to the fact that it can impede energy flow if tight and restrictive. In addition, all thoughts of previous clients and personal situations should be cleared from your mind to be able to focus your full attention.

- *Client* – removal and safekeeping of coats, jackets, briefcases, shopping etc. but keeping valuables e.g. handbags or wallet with them at all times.

Tip

If you feel comfortable shaking hands when you meet a new client, ensure that your handshake is firm and positive and your hands are clean and dry.

Introduction

An effective treatment relies on the interconnection between the client and practitioner so thought should be given to:

- *Greeting* – it is important to introduce yourself to the client positively, making full eye contact and speaking clearly and concisely using your tone of voice, choice of words and general body language in a welcoming manner.

- *Reference* – ensure that you are using the client's correct name and title, checking pronunciation as appropriate.
- *Process* – a first time client will have little or no knowledge of the treatment or of the consultation that precedes it. It is therefore necessary to spend a few moments discussing this to ensure that the client is comfortable with the processes and happy to proceed. Even regular clients need reminding of the process!

Remember

It takes a number of months to take on board the concepts of reflexology and gain your qualification. Remember this when you have a new client, and provide them with enough information to feed their curiosity and help them gain a healthy respect for you and the treatment without blinding them with science, causing unnecessary confusion.

Case history

An effective treatment relies on the efficient use of our senses and the examination may be classified as being **visual**, **oral**, **aural**, **olfactory**, **perceptive** and **tactile**:

- *Visual* – observe your client from the moment you greet them to the moment you leave them, taking note of what you see. Note a client's posture and general demeanour – what does this tell you about them? Note the way in which they walk to the treatment area and sit themselves down – was it difficult? Did they need assistance? Are they showing visual signs of nervousness? What is their breathing like? Do they visibly calm down during the consultation? This visual information will prove to be a vital aid to the development of the consultation.
- *Oral* – it will be necessary to ask questions and take note of the answers given. Be aware of the sensitivity of what is being said and reassure the client using your tone of voice as well as your choice of words. When discussing more personal information, a lack of embarrassment on your part will encourage the same attitude in the client. If the client is making a telephone enquiry, it may be necessary to take certain personal details from them other than their name and telephone number. If this is the case, check that the person is able to talk as they may feel inhibited if they are making the call from work etc.
- *Aural* – ensure that you are engaged in active listening, i.e. that you are both hearing and listening to what is being said. Use your body language to demonstrate to the client

that you are listening actively. Nod to confirm acknowledgement, smile to convey care, maintain eye contact to show interest etc.

- *Olfactory* – use your sense of smell to pick up further information from your client. The odour associated with the body generally, the feet and breath specifically may alert you to potential problem areas e.g. possible digestive disorders in the case of halitosis (foul-smelling breath), possible kidney problems in the case of foul smelling feet, etc. Be aware of the impression created with your own personal odour. Avoid the use of strong, heavy perfumes that may be off-putting for clients, paying particular attention to all aspects of your personal hygiene.

- *Perceptive* – you will intuitively get a sense of your client just as they will you. Be aware of your gut feeling – this will allow you to adapt your skills to suit the needs of the client more effectively. Be respectful of the client's sense of you. It may be that you are not the person to treat them – a consultation will provide them with the opportunity to decide this for themselves. We are in effect learning to read the client as much as they are trying to read their practitioner! As hard as we may try, we cannot be 'all things for all people'. There are many hundreds of reflexology practitioners – respect a client's need to test you out even if they do not ultimately choose you. Their freedom of choice will ensure that the practitioner they do choose is right for them at that time.

- *Tactile* – the use of touch is a necessary tool in advancing your consultation skills. It may be appropriate to touch the client to demonstrate that you empathise with them. It may be that the client's words touched you. Use the feelings that this evokes to create greater empathy, understanding and awareness of your client. The art of touch is the science of trust. Use touch sensitively and appropriately to get a feel for the person within.

Explanation

An efficient treatment relies on increasing knowledge and awareness on the part of the client. This encourages them to take an active role in the development of their own well-being, so thought should be given to providing the client with:

- *Treatment background* – it is useful to provide the client with some information relating to the history of the treatment. This may be done verbally or with the use of leaflets, posters, books etc.

- *Treatment procedure* – a client needs to know what the treatment entails e.g. which part of the body you are going to be treating, whether or not they need to remove any clothing, do they sit or lie down, if breathing exercises are to be carried out, how they will be conducted and when, that you may leave them to fetch a glass of water, wash your hands etc.

Tip

It is worth noting that different cultures and religions have different beliefs and the concept of reflexology may not be agreeable to everyone. It may be that after the initial explanation of the treatment a client realises that it is not for them. Their views must be respected.

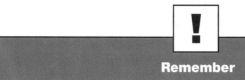

Remember

You will be comfortable with every aspect of the treatment and know exactly what will happen and when. Do not forget that the client does not have access to this information unless you tell them!

- *Effects and benefits* – it is important to make the client aware of what you can and cannot do. The information given should be realistic and accurate, ensuring that you avoid giving false hope.

Remember

You cannot make a medical diagnosis unless qualified to do so and you cannot cure a disorder. What you can do is provide a complement (with doctor's approval) and in some cases an alternative (for minor disorders e.g. stress-related) to medical treatment as well as help to stimulate the body's own healing and coping mechanisms.

Confirmation

When the necessary information has been discussed and recorded it is then possible to make a recommendation for treatment based on the client's needs. This recommendation is dependent on client approval and agreement and time must therefore be allocated within the consultation for client questions prior to their formal agreement of the proposed treatment. The treatment may then be booked for a specific date and time or, as in most cases, take place immediately after the consultation. Finally, both the client and the practitioner sign the consultation form:

- The client signs to agree the treatment but to also confirm that the information they have given is correct to the best of their knowledge and that they understand the implications of giving false information.
- The practitioner also signs to agree the treatment as well as to confirm that they have given correct information and recommendations regarding treatment to suit the client's individual needs as a result of the consultation process.

Tip

This information is important in the unlikely event of legal action being taken against the practitioner. A thorough consultation, which has been recorded and signed by both parties, demonstrates professionalism and is a sign of good practice.

Activity

Practise conducting stage one of the consultation on a partner using the consultation form as a guide. Adapt the form to provide yourself with a more personally user-friendly version. If you do not have enough knowledge of anatomy and physiology check Chapter 13 for details or refer to *An Holistic Guide to Anatomy and Physiology*.

Task 1

Experiment talking to someone when you are both seated at different heights. The person seated at the higher level automatically assumes a superior position and the person in the lower seat automatically feels inferior. Discuss with your partner how each position makes you feel.

Task 2

Make a list of at least three other resources you may want to have available to aid the consultation process and explain why.

Task 3

Draw up a checklist for personal presentation appropriate to your job role. Think about the importance of each aspect of the checklist.

Task 4

Draw up a security checklist relating to the safekeeping of client's belongings in your workplace. Alternatively, think about ways in which the current procedures used (if appropriate) can be improved.

Task 5

Devise a leaflet explaining the treatment that may be displayed in a reception area and/or sent out to clients who make telephone enquiries.

Consultation – stage two

9

The second stage of the consultation involves a physical examination of the area to be treated and is often referred to as reading the feet, hands or ears. It forms a continuation of the reading process that is carried out in stage one of the consultation. This reading of the feet, hands or ears is generally conducted as part of the treatment and is predominantly tactile incorporating the use of a technique called **palpation** in which pressure is applied with the fingers, thumbs and/or hand to feel the area being treated.

Tip

Palpation means the examination of a part by touch or pressure of the hand.

Visual, aural, olfactory and perceptive skills are also associated with stage two relating to what you see, hear, smell and sense. In addition, it may also be necessary to ask questions as well as discuss with the client the details of the examination. The information gained from this part of the consultation helps to confirm the information received during stage one.

Angel advice

Sometimes information that was not mentioned during stage one may come to light during stage two. It is important to treat this information sensitively, as it may be extremely sensitive in nature.

CONSULTATION STAGE TWO
PHYSICAL EXAMINATION

Right foot

Notes ....
....
....
....
....
....

Left foot

Notes ....
....
....
....
....
....

Right hand

Notes ....
....
....
....
....
....

Left hand

Notes ....
....
....
....
....
....

Right ear

Notes ....
....
....
....
....
....

Left ear

Notes ....
....
....
....
....

Angel advice

It is important to follow your own gut feeling as well as the guidelines.

Fascinating Fact

The study of the patterns of ridges of the skin of the palms of the hands and fingers and the soles of the feet and toes is known as **dermatoglyphics**. This is used as a means to establish the identity of a person both clinically and genetically in the interest of anthropology (the science of man) and law enforcement.

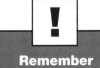

Remember

Yin is associated with the right hemisphere of the brain and as such the left side of the body. Yang is associated with the left hemisphere of the brain and as such the right side of the body.

Tip

The zones can be identified on the ears by linking the zones of the body with the position of the body as represented on the ear.

When conducting a physical examination it is useful to follow certain guidelines in terms of what to look for and the interpretation of such findings. Useful guidelines include **position**, **size** and **shape**, **colour**, **texture**, **temperature** and **conditions**.

Position

The position of the body part in relation to the whole body, i.e. on either the left or the right side, is believed to be associated with yin and yang, taking on the characteristics associated with each one.

- Right foot, hand or ear = yang. Associated with positive, active polarity, visual types, the past, male characteristics, physical aspects and energy from the sun. They are also associated with our relationships with men and the world in general as well as sympathetic nervous system activity (preparing for action) and assertive, analytical and logical actions.
- Left foot, hand or ear = yin. Associated with negative, inactive polarity, auditory types, the present, female characteristics, emotional aspects and energy from the earth. They are also associated with our relationships with women and our family as well as parasympathetic nervous system activity (preparing for rest) and nurturing, receptive and intuitive actions.

In addition the position of the smaller parts can be read in relation to the zones. This can be more easily identified in the feet and hands i.e.

- Big toes and thumbs = zone 1
- Second toes and index fingers = zone 2
- Third toes and middle fingers = zone 3
- Fourth toes and ring fingers = zone 4
- Little toes and fingers = zone 5.

Each zone is also believed to be represented by an element (Chapter 3), which can be further identified and read from the position of the fingers and toes.

- Big toes and thumbs = ether which has a yang association with joy and a yin association with sorrow.
- Second toes and index fingers = air which has a yang association with positive feelings and a yin association with negative feelings.
- Third toes and middle fingers = fire which has a yang association with logical thinking and a yin association with creative thinking.
- Fourth toes and ring fingers = water which has a yang association with attachment and a yin association with love.

- Little toes and fingers = earth which has a yang association with security and a yin association with trust.

Size and shape

The size and the shape of the part reflects the size and shape of the whole body i.e. it is generally recognised that a large person will have large feet, hands and ears etc. It then stands to reason that the corresponding mirrored body part will be of an equally proportioned size. Other factors may be considered:

- Position and shape of the waist and hip lines on the part reflects the position and shape of the waist and hips of the body i.e. high or low waisted, shapely waist and hips etc.

- A broad shape to the part often reflects a person with a broad body shape and a broad outlook, someone who is down to earth and practical in their approach to life.

- A narrow shaped part is often owned by a person with a narrow body shape and someone who likes to pay attention to the finer details in life. They may be described as being narrow minded.

- Straight and/or tight parts are often associated with a person who likes to set parameters. They often share a narrow shape to the part and the body as a whole and are regarded as the sort of person who likes to live life on the straight and narrow.

- Curvaceous and/or flexible parts reflect the body type as well as the kind of person who is more willing to bend or give.

Colour

The colour of the area to be treated will reflect both the physical and psychological condition of the part, the corresponding body part as well as the whole person, e.g.:

- Red – stimulated circulation to the area, a corresponding body part that has or is working excessively and stimulated emotions e.g. embarrassment, anger, frustration etc.

- White – poor circulation to the area, a corresponding body part that is overworked and possibly drained often accompanied by a general feeling of physical and emotional exhaustion.

- Blue/purple – bruised skin in the area, an associated body part that is tender and sore and perhaps bruised emotions.

- Yellow – possible kidney and/or liver problems together with the need for physical and emotional protection.

- Uneven colour – lack of balance caused by disturbed circulation which may manifest itself in a general loss of equilibrium to the part, the body and the mind.

Tip

Hard skin on the feet is often associated with poor posture, on the hands with hard manual work and on the ears with piercings, all reflecting excess pressure to the area and in turn the whole body.

Angel advice

What a person thinks about their feet, hands and/or ears reflects the way they think about themselves as a whole.

Texture

The texture of the skin will help to determine the condition of the body part, the mirrored part and the mind e.g.

- Rough skin – possible effects of the ageing process on the area and the corresponding body part as well as a person who may be experiencing a rough phase in their life.
- Hard skin – develops over an area for added protection, the associated body part may also be in need of special attention and the person may be feeling vulnerable and in need of extra care.
- Taut skin – tension in underlying muscles and associated body parts, the person may also be feeling strung up and stressed out.
- Flaking skin – lack of moisture to the area and associated body part and the person may be feeling generally irritable and out of sorts.
- Peeling skin – may signify a skin disorder e.g. athlete's foot, as well as a problem in the corresponding body part together with an emotional sign of releasing the old.
- Cracked skin – exposure to the elements, which has affected the part, the corresponding body part together with a general feeling of being torn apart.
- Puffiness – indicates general congestion which may be mirrored in the corresponding body part and reflected with feelings of overload.
- Grittiness – deposits of uric acid (often referred to as crystal deposits) are sometimes present at the end of capillaries as a result of cellular function and are felt as gritty lumps that can be tender to the touch. Their presence indicates a local build up of unreleased toxins, a possible build up in the corresponding body part together with a build up of unreleased emotions.

The condition of a client's feet, hands or ears will also reflect care and attention. If lack of care is evident of a part of the body then there is likely to be a lack of attention to the whole of the body! The possible causes of this will help to determine a person's mental state e.g.

- A lonely person may feel that as no one appears to care for them there is no reason why they should care for themselves.
- A person who has experienced physical/verbal abuse may have been made to feel that they do not deserve any care and so are afraid to care for themselves.
- A person who dislikes themself or a part of themself may feel that they are not worthy of care.

It is also worth noting that perhaps a person is not aware of how to take care of a certain part of their body and so needs specific advice on general aftercare e.g.

- Ensure the area is kept clean and dry.
- Exfoliate regularly using a product appropriate to the part e.g. facial scrub for ears (care should be taken to avoid the product entering the ears), body scrub for hands and feet.
- Moisturise daily to hydrate and protect the surface skin.
- Drink plenty of water to hydrate and protect from within.
- Pay attention to diet to ensure adequate nutrients are available for repair and maintenance.
- Pay attention to breathing to ensure that cellular respiration is efficient.
- Protect the area from the elements with suitable shoes, gloves and hats as appropriate. Ensure that these garments are comfortable, well fitted and do not restrict blood flow or cause excess pressure to the area.

Client care is therefore of primary importance during a consultation and can be a vital tool is encouraging the client to care for themselves.

Temperature

Normal body temperature is 36.8°C and is regulated by the activity in the blood vessels, skin and muscles, which is coordinated by the nervous system. In addition the activity of organs like those of digestion produce heat within the body. When the brain picks up on the fact that body temperature has changed it will alert the blood vessels to either conserve body heat by constricting surface blood capillaries or release excess heat by dilating surface capillaries. In addition to this the sweat glands are stimulated into producing sweat when body temperature rises and the formation of goose pimples and shivering occurs when the body temperature drops. Observing the temperature of the part can help to determine the activity in the rest of the body:

- *Warm* – if the part to be treated feels warm it signifies balance. It stands to reason that if there is localised balance then that should be reflected in the rest of the body and mind.
- *Hot* – if the part is hot to the touch the circulation has been stimulated and the increased blood to the area will be seen and the skin will appear red. This effect will be mirrored in corresponding areas of the body and mind where there will be an increase in activity.
- *Localised hot spots* – specific areas of stimulation relating to stimulation of specific areas of the body and mind.
- *Cold* – if the part feels cold, the circulation to the area is poor and the skin will appear pale. Corresponding areas of the body will reflect this lack of activity, as will the emotions, which may appear 'frozen'.
- *Localised cold spots* – lack of stimulation to specific areas of the parts will reflect lack of action in corresponding parts of the body and perhaps specific emotions.

Angel advice

Try to have an open mind when interpreting the results of what your senses pick up.

Remember

The effect of external irritation may affect the part – e.g. new shoes, earrings, finger and toe rings – the body takes time to adapt to such intrusions (sensory adaptation) and this should be taken into account when reading the part.

Remember

Note the possible causes of such conditions e.g. new shoes, pierced ears etc. and match your interpretations accordingly.

Conditions

Disorders that affect the part often have a knock-on effect on the corresponding body part as well as the whole body:

- Athlete's foot – can affect the whole foot and as a result a person may be experiencing physical and emotional irritation and frustration.
- Warts and verrucae – affect specific areas of the hands and feet and can signify the surfacing of specific physical and emotional problems.
- Blisters – caused by friction to the skin, may also signify physical and emotional friction.
- Split nails – nails are weak reflecting the physical and emotional well-being of the person as a whole.
- Ingrown nails – the nail grows back into the skin causing pain, which may reflect a person's physical and emotional state as they experience the need to withdraw within themselves.
- No nail – loss of nail due to injury or disease leaving the nail bed exposed and vulnerable which may mirror the way the person is feeling generally, both physically and emotionally.
- Inflamed skin – reflects the body's need to fight against attack, which may also be seen in inflamed emotions as a result of extreme aggravation.
- Infected skin – the result of attack on the body which may be seen as an open wound both physically and emotionally.
- Scars – the results of past physical and possibly emotional pain.

Tip

It is possible to track in all directions – what you see on the part may be mirrored in the body and mind – and certain circumstances will enable you to read the part before you read the person e.g. as part of a basic facial, Indian head massage; manicure or pedicure etc. In these situations your introductory consultation may not be as detailed as that required for reflexology. Alternatively, by reading the person first as in stage one of the reflexology consultation we can be alerted to how the outcomes e.g. symptoms, may manifest themselves as we read the part. This helps to confirm our prior reading.

Balanced position, size, shape, colour, texture, temperature and condition of the feet, hands and/or ears will reflect a balanced part which will give rise to a balanced body on all levels. Any deviation from this will be seen in physical, psychological and/or spiritual imbalance.

Activity

Practice conducting stage two of the consultation on a partner using the consultation form as a guide. Adapt the form to provide yourself with a more personally user-friendly version.

Once stages one and two of the consultation have been completed the treatment itself may take place. This forms a natural progression as the physical examination may be concluded with the relaxation techniques that are used to commence the treatment. Throughout the treatment examination of the area continues and notes are made accordingly on the relevant paperwork (Part 4 provides further detailed information).

Task 1

Look closely at the feet, hands and ears of yourself and/or a partner. Try to pick up on the differences between the left and right side. Think of each part in terms of yin and yang and try to link what you see with what you know of yourself and/or the other person.

Task 2

Try to identify your characteristics by examining the position, size and shape, colour, texture, temperature and conditions of your feet, hands and ears – can you recognise yourself? Do this with a partner and check your findings.

Task 3

For your own interest research different methods of reading the body e.g. Chinese face reading etc. Think of ways in which you can integrate different methods into your consultation.

Consultation – stage three

10

The third stage of the consultation involves the closing of the treatment, providing the opportunity to discuss outcomes, reactions, aftercare, home care and further treatments.

CONSULTATION STAGE THREE – TREATMENT CLOSE

Treatment date: ....

Outcomes: ....

....

....

Reactions: ....

....

....

Aftercare: ....

....

....

Homecare: ....

....

Further treatments: ....

....

....

Any other comments: ....

....

....

....

....

....

Angel advice

Once the practitioner has completed the manual treatment, it is advisable to leave the client for a few moments if possible. This provides the client with the opportunity to come to in their own time and space and allows the practitioner to disconnect from the treatment. The client may want to stretch out their body, rub their eyes, analyse their feelings etc. and will feel more comfortable doing so on their own. The practitioner can wash their hands, fetch themselves and the client a glass of water, and gather their thoughts and focus for the closing of the treatment. If the client has been lying down it is important that they resume a seated position for the close of the treatment to ensure eye contact can be maintained at an equal level.

Outcomes

Giving and obtaining feedback is a vital part of the treatment, providing the practitioner and the client with the means to find out more about how the treatment relates to the individual, for example:

- It is necessary to discuss your findings with the client, relating them to the information gained at each stage of the consultation.
- It is also useful to obtain feedback from the client with reference to how they felt during the treatment, discussing their individual experiences as well as how they are feeling post-treatment.
- It is useful for subsequent treatments to ask the client to record their feelings both physically and emotionally over the next 24–48 hours.

Reactions

A client needs to be aware of the type of reactions they may realistically expect to experience as a result of the treatment they have received. The possible reactions are dependent on the condition of the client prior to treatment and the type of treatment given – length of treatment and depth of pressure etc. The common reactions to treatment may be classified in terms of output or release and input or replenish and may be experienced up to 48-hours post-treatment.

As a result of stimulating the body systems through reflexology treatment a client may reasonably expect to experience some form of release:

- This may take the form of an increased need to urinate. Urine may be darker and stronger smelling.
- There may be an increase in bowel movements with possible accompanying flatulence.
- An increase in vaginal discharge may occur together with greater blood flow during menstruation as the body undergoes a clearing process.
- Increased mucus secretions in the nose, mouth and throat.
- In certain circumstances even sweating and flu-like symptoms may occur post-treatment.
- Skin breakouts, especially when conditions have been suppressed.
- Aching muscles and headaches may occur as a natural reaction to the release of excessive physical and mental tension and stress.
- The release of emotions is a natural process in the healing of the mind and a client may experience a heightening of feelings such as agitation, anger, laughter, weeping etc. as a result.

These are all natural releasing processes which form a part of the body's own healing mechanisms.

Remember

Sleep is the body's way of natural rejuvenation.

It may be that post-treatment the body needs to replenish itself in some way, and the client may experience the need for some form of input:

- Increased feelings of hunger and/or thirst may accompany the close of a treatment as a more relaxed mind is alerted to the body's need for nutrients.

- A natural response to reflexology is one of tiredness through to extreme exhaustion post-treatment as the body attempts to make the person aware of its need for sleep.

- Feelings of emptiness often accompany the release of extreme emotions and this is often followed by the need to be nurtured and cared for. The reflexology treatment helps to fulfil these needs as well as to encourage a person to take more care of themselves.

These natural reactions may be referred to as **contra actions** and are often viewed as being part of a '**healing crisis**'. A contra action is most commonly classified as an adverse reaction to treatment and may be characterised as a disturbance of state. We get used to living and feeling a certain way and do not always realise the effects this has on our state of balance until alerted to them through treatments such as reflexology. A healing crisis refers to a turning point or danger point and may be seen as an extreme reaction to treatment. It is characterised by the body's need to get worse before it gets better. Many people put illness on hold until a convenient time or until their body cannot hold out any longer. Think about the type of people who say that they do not have time to be ill and/or are only ill when they have time off work e.g. weekends and holidays. A reflexology treatment encourages the body to activate its own healing and coping mechanisms by stimulating the body systems to work together more harmoniously. As a result a person is forced to respond to the reactions. Sometimes the coping mechanisms have been exhausted and the only way the body can activate its healing mechanisms is to allow a period of time for input and replenishment. The more balanced a person becomes these reactions realistically lessen and a state of equilibrium is more readily achievable.

 Case study

I have a client, a very high-powered businessman who decided to 'try out' foot reflexology a few years ago. During the consultation he insisted on telling me that everything in his body was fine and that he was never ill. On observing his body language and reading his feet I was not sure that I agreed with his description of himself. As I started the treatment I intuitively felt that he was experiencing symptoms of extreme

▶

Case study *(continued)*

exhaustion and it very quickly came to light that his body needed help. Although the treatment I gave was extremely light he began to feel dizzy and faint and we stopped the treatment and discussed his reactions. He had been experiencing symptoms of excessive stress in the form of panic attacks and inability to sleep for some time but had chosen to ignore them. The reflexology treatment had in effect forced him to face up to the fact that he was unable to cope in his current state and encouraged him to admit that he was in need of special care. As a result he decided to take time out of work to reassess his situation and allow his body time to readjust. Four years on he now enjoys regular reflexology treatments with no adverse reactions, and has a more realistic view of life and his place within it.

Angel advice

One of the most important outcomes of the treatment is increased awareness, which should be acted upon if healing is to take place. The old saying 'you can take a horse to water but you cannot make it drink' is very apt. You can make a person aware of their body and what it needs through treatment but you cannot make them respond. It is up to each individual to take responsibility for their own well-being by listening to their body and taking the appropriate action.

Angel advice

How many times have we heard people saying that they haven't had the time to go to the loo during the course of a day? Think about the accumulative adverse affects this has on the body and mind as the body fills up with unreleased waste! This thought alone is enough to remind us to go!

Aftercare

It is not only important to alert a client to the likely reactions to treatment but also to what action they should take, for example:

- Respond to the releasing requirements of the body i.e. fulfil the urge to urinate, defecate etc. Allow time for the body to activate its healing mechanisms and consider ways in which the coping mechanisms may be enhanced by avoiding excesses.

- Respond to the replenishing requirements of the body i.e. natural, uncarbonated spring water and a light meal is recommended post-treatment. The avoidance of caffeine, alcohol and foods that are difficult to digest is advisable. A period of rest is recommended post-treatment with any further activity monitored to ensure that any excess is avoided where possible.

Tip

Justification of a proposed course of aftercare promotes greater understanding and in turn more action!

Angel advice

The key to balance and harmony lies in achieving a balance between input and output.

Remember

It often takes people a long time to become stressed and/or ill. In the same way it will also take time for a person to become de-stressed and/or well. Neither situation happens overnight.

Aftercare is usually basic common sense, but it should still be reinforced as part of the consultation process for all clients.

Home care

In addition to basic aftercare advice, information should be available for the client to continue caring for themselves between treatments. This advice should be relevant to the information gained during the consultation and treatment, achievable for the client and within the limits of the practitioner's expertise. Home care advice may include information on the following (see Part 4 for more details relating to each body system):

- Nutrition – basic advice relating to healthy breathing, eating and drinking.
- Ageing – information on the effects of ageing and realistic techniques to help to counteract and accept this process.
- Rest and activity – the importance of achieving balance and harmony.
- Awareness – listening to the body and responding accordingly.
- Special care – realistic self-help techniques to de-stress.

Home care should be individual to each client and form the basis for continued self-development, remembering to refer a client to a specialist when recommendations are out of the realms of your expertise. This encourages clients to take responsibility for their own well-being.

Further treatments

Advice can be given on subsequent and complementary treatments. Holistic treatments such as reflexology offer cumulative effects over a period of time and care should be taken to explain this to a client, relating the timing to the nature and severity of their condition.

There is no limit to how often a reflexology treatment may be carried out but certain guidelines should be adhered to in terms of:

- Length of treatment – actual treatment time is usually between 25–35 minutes plus consultation time. Less time is required the more often the treatment is carried out i.e. daily treatment would be shorter than weekly treatment to avoid overstimulation.
- Depth of treatment – the amount of pressure applied depends on the area to be treated and attention should be paid to the results of the consultation to ensure that discomfort is kept to a minimum e.g. a client suffering with diarrhoea will suffer with a tender abdominal region. Treatment of the corresponding area on the feet, hands and/or ears should be light and soothing to avoid excessive

Angel advice

It is nice to complete this stage with a final thought that in effect ties up the whole treatment. This can be done in a variety of ways e.g. by asking the client to pick an affirmation card at random whilst focusing on a particular aspect of the treatment outcome.

discomfort, unnecessary contra actions and possible further aggravation.

● Frequency of treatment – treatment may be carried out daily, weekly or monthly depending on the needs of the client and their circumstances. A general guide to follow would be weekly treatments over a period of a month to gain a greater insight into the client and their conditions. The results can then be reviewed and a further plan of treatment reassessed accordingly.

It may be necessary to provide a client with advice on other treatments that complement reflexology so that they can gain maximum benefit from holistic care (see Chapter 4, A–Z of Complementary Therapies for reference). If you are unable to perform these treatments, ensure that suitable recommendations and referrals are made.

The close of the consultation provides the time for any final client questions and confirms the ending with the completion of payment and subsequent booking details.

Activity

Use your imagination and think of interesting ways to provide your clients with a positive memory to sum up the consultation/treatment and one that will have a lasting effect until their next visit. In this way clients will often say that they feel the presence of their practitioner, likening it to 'a little voice over my shoulder' providing comfort and guidance long after the treatment has taken place.

Task 1

Devise a client questionnaire to be used by the client post treatment. Include questions relating to the treatment as well as how they felt over the next 24–48 hours. Think about how you can use the information gained in subsequent treatments.

Task 2

Devise a general aftercare sheet that may be given to the client during stage three of the consultation. Refer to Part 4 for specific care of body systems.

11

Business matters

The consultation should be conducted in a caring and professional manner with attention being paid to industry **codes of ethics** as well as **legislative requirements**.

Codes of ethics

This is a specific set of rules laid down by a regulatory body to safeguard the welfare of the reflexology client and the reflexology practitioner, including:

- Conduct – professional working methods observing client confidentiality and privacy whilst maintaining moral and hygienic codes of practice.

Remember

When treating members of the opposite sex it is important not to do so alone. Ensure someone else is within ear shot to safeguard both you and the client against any possible misinterpretation of treatment.

- Practice – professional working area and practice should be maintained at all times adapted to suit the circumstances e.g. working within a client's home etc.
- Referral – clients with conditions beyond the limits of the practitioner's expertise should be referred to a suitable and reputable specialist and any subsequent reflexology treatment should be with the appropriate specialist's approval.
- Record keeping – information collected from the client should be dealt with sensitively and securely. Access to

record cards should be restricted to the practitioner. Clients are able to read their own records on request.

- Insurance – public liability (refers to damage to the client whilst in your establishment) and professional indemnity (refers to damage caused to a client during treatment) are not statutory requirements but are necessary when a practitioner joins a regulatory body.

- Qualifications – recognised qualifications are a requirement of all responsible regulatory bodies and demonstrate that a certain level of competency has been achieved. Providing clients with access to view your qualifications is good practice, as is inclusion in recommended lists forwarded to clients from recognised organisations.

- Continued Professional Development (CPD) – there is a constant need to update and progress the direct skills associated with reflexology and the indirect skills associated with other holistic treatments, business management etc. Life-long learning is the key to any treatment provision and time should be allocated to ensure that this takes place on a regular basis. Activities may include sharing experiences with other practitioners, attending trade fairs, exhibitions and reading trade magazines, experiential learning through giving and receiving treatments, formal training for recognised qualifications, informal workshops, staff meetings etc.

Legislative requirements

A general set of rules laid down by a government department to safeguard the health, safety and welfare of the general public (clients and practitioners – employed and self-employed) including:

- The Health and Safety at Work Act 1974 (HASAWA) – the environment in which the reflexology treatment is to take place must conform to certain guidelines e.g. safe equipment and safe systems of work, safe handling, storage and transport of substances, safe place of work with safe entrance and exit, adequate facilities and protective equipment.

- The Work Place (health, safety and welfare) Regulations 1992 – this relates to the maintenance of the workplace and equipment in terms of ventilation, temperature, lighting, cleanliness, sanitary and washing facilities, supply of drinking water and safety of personal belongings.

- Health and Safety (first aid) Regulations 1981 – employers should provide adequate facilities for administering first aid. When working alone it is good practice to have access to a first aid box for minor first aid problems and to be a trained first aider in the event of more serious problems.

- The Working Time Regulations 1998 – regulates the number of hours worked by an employed person. Self-employed people have no such restrictions but should

Tip

The working temperature of a room should be maintained at approximately 16°C or 61°F.

Angel advice

Better to be safe than sorry!

Tip

Always check the ingredients in any product you purchase or use to ensure that they comply with these regulations. If in doubt – avoid use!

Tip

Fire precautions must be observed if candles are used in the consultation/treatment area to create a calming ambience.

monitor their working time in accordance with their stress levels and health.

● The Management of Health and Safety at Work Regulations 1999 – recommends the assessment of the risks to staff and clients whilst undertaking or receiving treatment. Such assessments should thereby reduce the risks and have procedures in place in the event of a problem occurring.

● Control of Substances Hazardous to Health Regulations 1999 (COSHH) – any substance that can be inhaled, ingested and/or absorbed into the skin must be identified and assessed for risks to health. As a result, substances should be appropriately labelled, effective measures employed to reduce any risks and any possible risks regularly reviewed e.g. clients with nut allergies are at risk if products containing nut extracts are used on them. Appropriate questions should be asked during stage one of the consultation and alternative products made available.

● The Dangerous Substances and Preparations (nickel) Regulations 2000 – this prohibits the use of products containing nickel or nickel compound which may come into contact with the skin unless the rate of nickel release is less than 0.5 microgrammes per week.

● Employers Liability (compulsory insurance) Act 1969 – if you employ staff it is your responsibility to ensure that you are insured against liability for injury or disease sustained in the course of employment. An employer must insure for at least £5 million for any individual claim and a certificate of insurance must be displayed. This ruling applies to work experience students also.

● Electricity at Work Act 1989 – it is necessary to list all electrical items used as part of the supply of any treatment including CD players, kettles etc. These items should be checked prior to use, adequately maintained and tested by an outside contractor yearly. Results of electrical testing must be recorded.

● The Reporting of Injuries, Diseases and Dangerous Occurrences Regulations 1995 **RIDDOR** – notification of major injury or disease must be made to the Incident Contact Centre. In addition, an accident report book should be available to record accidents and injury.

● The Fire Precautions Act 1971 – a fire certificate is required if more than twenty people are employed on one floor, or more than ten people on different floors at any one time. All premises should have adequate fire fighting equipment and access to escape in the event of a fire. Fire extinguishers should be checked annually and training provided for safe use.

● The Environmental Protection Act 1990 – care should be taken in the safe disposal of waste by following manufacturer's guidelines. It is good practice to dispose of waste such as couch roll and tissues in a double bin bag.

- The Provisions and Use of Work Equipment Regulations 1992 – all equipment must be suitable for use, properly maintained and appropriate training undertaken prior to use.

- Personal Protective Equipment at Work Regulations 1992 – personal protection should be considered when using products or equipment that expose a person to any possible risk.

- The Health and Safety Display Screen Equipment Regulations 1992 – it is commonly recognised that excessive computer work can lead to eye strain, mental and physical stress. To avoid this, use should be limited to safe timings. This is useful advice for clients who may not have employers to monitor safe use as well as for ourselves.

- Manual Handling Operations Regulations 1992 – safety procedures for manual handling to prevent injury. Care should be taken to avoid lifting anything that is too heavy, ensure that any lifting is carried out with bent knees and a straight back, and not to carry heavy loads too far or for too long.

- Trade Descriptions Act 1968 and 1972 – to avoid making any false allegations as to the effects and benefits of the treatments and/or products used.

- The Consumer Protection Act 1987 – to safeguard against the sale and use of unsafe products and services.

- The Sale and Supply of Goods Act 1994 – prevents the sale of goods and/or services that are defective and do not meet recognised standards.

- Data Protection Act 1984 – any business that stores information relating to staff and/or clients on a computer must register with the Data Protection Registrar. This is not a necessary requirement for manual records.

- Sex Discrimination Act 1975 and 1986 – ensures equal opportunities for all employees. Good practice ensures that clients of differing sexual orientation are not disadvantaged in anyway.

- Race Relations Act 1976 – ensures equal opportunities relating to race. Good practice ensures that clients of all races are treated with sensitivity and tact and that care is taken to respect any cultural differences.

- The Disability Discrimination Act 1995 – the working environment should provide adequate access and facilities to prevent staff and clients with disabilities from being disadvantaged.

In addition to the legislative requirements, the following are considerations when treating members of the public:

- Local authority licence – it is necessary to register your business with the local council and abide by any byelaws they enforce.

● Performing Rights Society (PRS) – it is illegal to play copyrighted music in an area open to the general public unless a fee is paid annually to the PRS. Some companies supply non-copyrighted music which is exempt from such requirements.

As well as adhering to a code of ethics and legislative requirements it is also good practice to have a prepared policy statement for the following:

● Health and safety – general guidelines that demonstrate the thought and action given to the welfare of clients and staff.

● Hygiene – a checklist for clients and staff to measure performance.

● Equal opportunities – a formal commitment to fair provision of service.

● Complaints procedure – a formal means by which clients and staff can address any problems they may encounter.

Finally, a consultation may be seen as a connecting process between the client, practitioner and treatment and as a result, has the potential be either **effective** or **non-effective**.

● An effective consultation involves intuitive practice set amongst a backdrop of theory (rules, regulations and guidelines) to ensure health, safety and welfare resulting in an open dialogue between client and practitioner for the good of the treatment.

● A non-effective consultation is one that ignores the balance between theory and practice, becoming either impersonal and automated or too personal and inappropriate.

As with all things holistic, care should be taken to ensure that there is balance and harmony between the opposing elements, in this case the theory and the practice of the consultation process. Paying attention to the theory ensures that the consultation is carried out correctly; being aware that the practice can be adapted ensures that the consultation feels right.

Tip

It is useful to get involved with local initiatives associated with small businesses that may be able to provide additional support and access to information e.g. local business clubs etc.

Task 1

It is advisable to carry out a risk assessment on the premises you will be working from and the products and tools you will be working with to ensure that all health, safety and welfare rules have been observed. Make a list of the potential dangers e.g. tripping on the stairs or possible allergies from products etc. Assess the risk factors – high, medium or low – and describe the necessary actions e.g. use of first aider/first aid box, sensitivity testing etc.

Task 2

Research your responsibilities under the codes of ethics and legislative requirements. You can obtain further information from your college, workplace, local authority or regulatory bodies such as HABIA. Alternatively review the codes of practice in your workplace and make suggestions for improvement where appropriate.

Task 3

It may be common practice in some professional organisations to adopt a set format for consultations. Make a list of the possible restrictions that might be imposed if you had to conduct a consultation to a set formula i.e. use the same set of questions in the same order for every client who visits for a reflexology treatment.

Task 4

Start to compile a portfolio of evidence to demonstrate your commitment to provision of service. Include all paperwork that may be used during the consultation e.g. consultation forms, information sheets, client questionnaires, aftercare sheets. Also include information relating to the health, safety and welfare of the clients relating to the code of ethics and legislative requirements e.g. qualification certificates, insurance documents, policy statements etc. This portfolio may be added to as you progress and provides a focal point for client information.

Part 4

The treatment

Learning objectives

After reading this part you should be able to:

- **Recognise the systems of the body and corresponding areas on the feet, hands and ears.**

- **Identify the specific reflex points on the feet, hands and ears.**

- **Understand the links between the condition of the reflex points and the symptoms associated with the corresponding body parts.**

- **Be aware of the factors that relate to the stimulation of each reflex point in terms of consultation, treatment and aftercare considerations.**

- **Begin to appreciate and make use of all of the skills required to undertake a reflexology treatment for the relief of stress and stress-related problems.**

Stress and reflexology

12

The reflexology treatment itself can take place once a thorough consultation has been completed, taking into account the skills discussed in the previous chapters.

As a result of an effective consultation the practitioner is able to agree a suitable course of action with the client. The main priority of such action is the relief of **stress**. Stress can be described as being 'the pressure associated with any factor (physical, psychological or spiritual) which can adversely affect the functioning of the body as a whole and which has the potential to disturb natural **homeostasis**'.

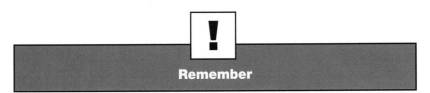

Remember

Homeostasis refers to the natural balance and stability of the body, mind and spirit needed for health.

The nature of stress

Stress is a fact of life and has been since time began. Our ancient ancestors faced the stresses associated with basic survival e.g. protection and provision, and as the earth and its inhabitants have evolved so has the nature of stress. Whilst the human body is equipped to cope with a certain amount of stress and strain it strives for balance and equilibrium and as such a burst of energy needs to be counteracted by a time of rest. Stress initiates a set of actions within the body that enable it to cope with the functions required of it, i.e. to face the stress head on (fight) or to run away from the stress (flight) hence the term 'fight or flight'.

Remember

Endocrine glands secrete their substances (hormones) directly into the blood supply for transport to the appropriate cells to initiate changes within the body.

Tip

Adrenalin is a stress hormone and is known as the 'fight or flight' hormone, preparing the body for increased physical and mental exertion.

Tip

Noradrenalin is a neurotransmitter of the sympathetic nervous system and exerts the same effects as adrenalin in preparation for fight or flight.

The fight or flight response

- A stressful situation is picked up by the body through the special sense organs – the ears, eyes, nose, skin and tongue – or internally through the nervous system itself.
- These sense organs alert the brain which in turn activates the hypothalamus that links the two controlling systems (nervous and endocrine) of the body to release corticotrophin-releasing hormone (CRH).
- CRH stimulates the pituitary gland (the master endocrine gland in the brain) to release adrenocorticotrophic hormone (ACTH) which stimulates the outer cortex of the adrenal glands.
- The adrenal cortex in turn increases the release of the hormone **cortisol**.
- At the same time the hormones **adrenalin** and **noradrenalin** are released from the inner medulla of the adrenal glands in response to stimuli from the sympathetic nervous system.
- Prolonged stress causes continued cortisol, adrenalin and noradrenalin release.

The effects of cortisol are that it:

- Helps to maintain resistance to stress.
- Allows adrenalin and noradrenalin to exert their effect.
- Inhibits immune activity.
- Prevents the body from over-responding to stress e.g. suppresses inflammation.

The effects of adrenalin and noradrenalin are:

- Increased blood flow to brain to improve mental activity.
- Increased blood flow to muscles to improve muscle strength and endurance.
- Increased levels of breathing to improve oxygen intake.
- Conversion of glycogen in the liver for an additional energy source.
- Reduced blood flow to digestive and urinary organs, slowing down digestion and the release of waste.
- Increased sweating to reduce body temperature.

Stress and health

Nowadays our basic survival needs are well catered for and within our culture it is generally accepted that we do not have to fight to protect ourselves or take flight when faced with a wild animal whilst hunting for food! However, modern day stresses can feel as threatening as those faced by our ancestors and initiate the same responses within the body. Health problems arise when the times of stress are not counteracted by times of calm and when stress becomes excessive and continuous. Stress may be characterised as being **safe** and **unsafe**.

Safe stress

Enables us to function at optimum levels. It provides us with the impetus to get motivated, to be positive and to achieve against adversity. It may be *seen* as the means of following a dream, *felt* as a driving force and *heard* as a little voice within providing a means of inner encouragement and guidance. It is also associated with stimulated energy flow and may be described as the 'X' factor that makes us stand out from the crowd. Safe stress has the power to promote action but as with all power it needs to be regularly refuelled. Refuelling can only be achieved if there is balance within the body and this can only occur if all of its needs are being met e.g. through breathing, drinking, eating, sleeping, relaxation etc.

Safe stress, therefore results in a cessation of the release of cortisol, adrenalin and noradrenalin once a stressful situation has passed, allowing the body to return to normal. Safe stress sees the calming of energy flow after a period of stimulation.

Unsafe stress

Occurs when the balance is uneven and the power and use of energy outweighs the refuelling and regenerating time. Modern day living is responsible for this imbalance and times when a person has to use more power and has less time to refuel can be identified in most people's lifetime. Such situations include:

- The death of a loved one.
- The birth of a baby.
- The breakdown of a relationship.
- Loss of job or redundancy.
- Moving house.
- Changing job role.
- Starting something new e.g. training course.
- Meeting new people.
- Environmental factors e.g. noise, pollution etc.

Unsafe stress, therefore, results in prolonged release of cortisol, adrenalin and noradrenalin, causing problems associated with the overuse of the body systems involved with coping with stress.

The way in which the body responds to stress is known as the general adaptation syndrome (GAS) and follows set stages including **alarm reaction**, **resistance** and finally **exhaustion**.

Activity

Make a list of at least five more examples of unsafe stress and think about the physical and psychological effects they may have on a person.

Fascinating Fact

A syndrome is a group of symptoms which frequently occur together and form a distinctive disease.

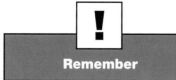

Remember

Acute refers to diseases which are sudden, severe and short in duration whilst diseases which are classed as being chronic are of a longer duration and more severe and debilitating.

Fascinating Fact

Statistics show that approximately 70 per cent of modern day diseases are the result of unsafe stress e.g. high blood pressure, migraines, hay fever, allergies, skin disorders, irritable bowel syndrome, etc.

Angel advice

Many people experiencing the effects of unsafe stress rely on the use of avoidance techniques, turning to alcohol, smoking, drugs, exercise etc. as a means of short-term relief. Such behaviour results in a further threat to health if it becomes excessive and obsessive.

1. Alarm reaction – an initial stressful situation sets off the fight or flight response with the secretion of adrenalin and noradrenalin. This is the body's way of coping by putting into place a set of actions to counteract the potential adverse effects imposed by the stressor. This manifests itself in a set of symptoms which we commonly recognise as being associated with a stressful situation – butterflies in the stomach, trembling, hot and clammy hands, racing heart beat and quick, shallow breathing.

2. Resistance – the secretion of cortisol, which is slower acting and longer lasting than adrenalin and noradrenalin, maintains a resistance to stress, helping to regulate the body's responses. As a result the organs and body systems involved with combating stress come under increasing pressure and start to weaken and the body experiences a set of symptoms commonly associated with prolonged stress – headaches, aching muscles, loss of appetite, lethargy and difficulty sleeping etc. A tendency to be more susceptible to acute conditions such as diarrhoea, colds, thrush and cystitis often accompany this stage as the body's immunity is weakened.

3. Exhaustion – continuous secretion of cortisol accompanies long-term stress. This results in a gradual weakening of the organs and body systems responsible for coping with and resisting stress. The body gradually loses its defence mechanisms and a state of exhaustion develops as cells are unable to regenerate. This stage is associated with chronic and degenerative illness, as homeostasis can no longer be maintained – migraines, diabetes, high blood pressure etc.

Therefore long-term, unsafe stress and the resulting general adaptation syndrome force the body and mind to experience changes resulting in greater susceptibility to **disease, wear and tear, ageing, neuroses** and **psychoses**:

- Disease – as a result of unsafe stress and lowered immunity the body is more prone to illness and disease.

- Wear and tear – like a machine, the body will suffer adverse effects as a result of overuse and lack of care.

- Ageing – time waits for no man or woman and passes irrespectively. This passing of time exerts its own pressures on the ageing process, which is further aggravated by the debilitating effects of unsafe stress.

- Neuroses – normal thoughts or feelings are exaggerated to such a degree that they adversely affect the sufferer's everyday life e.g. anxiety, hysteria, phobias, obsessions and depression.

- Psychoses – derangement of the personality resulting in loss of contact with reality e.g. manic depression, recurrent severe depression and schizophrenia.

Stress and well-being

Stress is an holistic phenomena affecting the whole body and as such has the potential to threaten its total well-being. The alarm stage associated with the general adaptation syndrome provides the body with an early warning system. Failure to respond to the associated symptoms initiates the next stage as resistance to stress builds up and symptoms of acute disease develop. Ignoring these symptoms puts the body at risk further as symptoms increase and disease becomes chronic in nature. The degeneration that follows eventually results in death.

If, along the way, the warning signs are acted upon, the body can enforce restorative mechanisms that are known as self-healing. During childhood, the care of a person's well-being is the responsibility of the parent. During adulthood the responsibility gradually shifts as each individual develops the necessary skills to manage their own well-being. Unfortunately, these skills are often taken for granted and failure to notice the warning signs that the body puts out when stress levels become dangerously high frequently occurs. Just as the body takes time to go through the degenerative changes associated with disease, it also takes time to go through the healing stages associated with well-being. To lead a healthy life there should be balance between all opposing forces and in an ideal world, for every stressful situation one faces, a counteracting calming situation should follow. This balance allows the body's healing mechanisms to be activated, helping to restore health and well-being.

Stress and reflexology

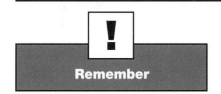

Remember

The word **holistic** comes from the Greek word **holos** meaning whole.

We do not live in an ideal world and it is important to put into place strategies that help one to cope effectively with the stresses and strains of everyday life. Reflexology provides one such strategy treating the body holistically.

By drawing on the information gained during the consultation and recognising that the body is made up of a sum of its parts, the practitioner is able to treat the whole person rather than just a symptom.

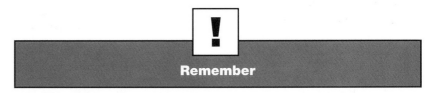

Remember

Homeostasis results in well-being which cannot be maintained unless all the parts of the body are working in harmony with one another. A symptom is a sign that all is not well within the body. Therefore a part of the body cannot be well unless the whole of the body is well.

Reflexology helps to:

- Identify stress-related symptoms through the consultation process.
- Associate areas of stress with corresponding symptoms through examination of the feet, hands and/or ears e.g. colour, texture, shape etc.
- Highlight areas of stress at each stage of the general adaptation syndrome through treatment to the feet, hands and/or ears.
- Isolate and treat specific areas of stress through the direct reflexes as mapped out on the feet, hands and/or ears e.g. the direct reflex associated with vomiting would be the stomach as this is the area *directly* affected.
- Discover and treat areas of stress associated with a recognised disorder through indirect or associated reflexes e.g. other parts of the body are going to be affected as a result of the body experiencing vomiting i.e. oesophagus, throat, mouth, muscles etc. which are all associated with the physical action.
- Track associated areas of stress through the zones and meridians e.g. if a problem has been identified in a part of a zone or meridian, the rest of the zone or meridian will be affected due to the blockage in energy flow.
- Track associated areas of stress through the links with the body systems e.g. if the muscles surrounding the spine are tense, the nerve impulses to and from the peripheral nerves are impeded, affecting the supply to and from the muscles of the rest of the body etc.
- Track associated areas of stress through the chakra system e.g. the sacral area of the spine relates to the sacral chakra. Backache experienced in this area will have an effect on energy flow within the chakra and corresponding body parts.
- Work cross-reflexes in the event of a contraindication preventing or restricting treatment e.g. work the hands instead of the feet, treat the shoulder reflex for the hip reflex etc.
- Activate self-healing by reducing stress hormone secretion, thus allowing the body to return to a stress-free state.
- Introduce balance and harmony to the body systems through treatment to each organ and the body systems as a whole.

Tip

Cross-reflexes may also be classified as referral reflexes or zones.

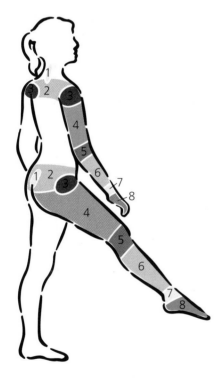

1 Cervical vertebrae – sacrum and coccyx
2 Shoulder girdle – pelvic girdle
3 Shoulder joint – hip joint
4 Upper arm – thigh
5 Elbow – knee
6 Forearm – lower leg
7 Wrist – ankle
8 Hand – foot

Cross reflexes

In addition reflexology helps a person to become more in tune with their body, encouraging them to listen to the warning signs, putting them in a better position to activate their own healing mechanisms to bring about a restored state of well-being.

With all of this in mind, care should be taken to ensure that both the client and the practitioner enjoy a stress free treatment and thought should therefore be given to the preparation of the **environment, equipment, tools, practitioner** and **client**.

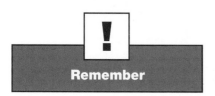

Tip

It is also useful to stay within sight of a clock to check treatment timing.

Remember

To observe the relevant health and safety guidelines when using candles.

Environment

It is usual to transfer the client from the seated position necessary to conduct a consultation to a more relaxed position for the treatment itself. In addition, the lights may be dimmed, suitable music switched on, a candle lit and maybe the use of an oil burner with a suitable oil – all of which change the formal setting associated with a consultation to a more tranquil setting which is conducive to treatment having a calming effect on the visual and auditory aspects of the brain (left and right).

Tip

Essential oils in an oil burner must be used with care, ensuring that the client finds the aroma agreeable.

The position of the client and practitioner should ensure comfort as well as adequate access to the working area i.e. feet, hands or ears.

- For foot reflexology the practitioner sits at the foot of the client. The client may be seated with their legs outstretched and supported on a couch or stool or alternatively the client may be totally or semi-reclined.
- For hand reflexology the practitioner and client may sit opposite, next to or diagonal to one another resting the hands on a table and/or pillow for support.
- For ear reflexology the client may be seated or reclined with the practitioner working behind or to the side in a standing or seated position.

Angel advice

Whichever position is adopted by the client and practitioner the emphasis must be on safety, comfort and access.

Equipment

The type of equipment used is dependent on availability and access and a treatment need not be hindered if the perfect couch and trolley etc. are not freely available. The treatment can be adapted to suit the equipment available, for example ear reflexology may be carried out with the client seated on the floor and the practitioner seated on a stool, foot reflexology may be carried out with the client seated in a comfy armchair with their feet resting on a footstool whilst the practitioner sits on the floor, hand reflexology may be carried out with the client lying on a bed and the practitioner seated on the bed etc.

Additional items that should be available include:

- Pillows – to rest the head, hands or feet for extra comfort.
- Towels – rolled up to provide support under the ankles, knees, neck etc.
- Blanket/duvet – for the client to lay/sit on and/or to cover the client for additional warmth and comfort.
- Disposable tissue roll – protective covering for couch/chair/trolley/table surfaces.
- Covered bin with bin liner – to hold any waste e.g. tissues etc.

Products

It is generally accepted that a reflexology treatment is carried out without the use of any products. It is thought that the use of oils or creams creates a barrier to the treatment, preventing the isolation of specific reflex points.

However, the use of products may be applied to perform the relaxation movements at both the start and end of the reflexology treatment. This aids relaxation as the practitioner can perform the movements with greater ease and to greater effect if incorporated with a massage medium. Suitable massage mediums include **oil**, **cream** or **talc**:

- Oil – may be used for a drier skin type and/or for longer relaxation time when extra slip is needed to perform the required movements.
- Cream – may be used for all skin types providing nourishment and a certain amount of slip needed to perform relaxation movements.
- Talc – this is used for a more greasy and/or sweaty skin type as it helps to absorb any excess moisture, preventing slip when working specific reflex points where accurate precision is required.

Additional products that should be made available include antiseptic wipes or sprays which may be used to cleanse the area to be treated as well as cleanse the practitioner's hands if access to running water is limited.

Practitioner

As the reflexology process progresses from consultation to treatment the practitioner should remain focused and constantly aware of the client's physical and psychological needs. Adaptation of body language and tone of voice should accompany the transition from the consultation, which is more formal and informative, to the treatment, which is more informal and intuitive.

Tip

Any excess product may be removed with warm mitts or alternatively a spritzer-type spray.

Tip

Care should be taken when using talc to avoid over use and the associated risks of inhalation of the fine particles. Cornflour or talc-free powder may be used as an alternative. The particles are less irritating to the respiratory system if inhaled.

Angel advice

The comfort of the practitioner is equally important and care should be taken to ensure correct posture is maintained throughout the application of the treatment to avoid excessive stress and strain.

Client

Preparation of the client needs to ensure maximum levels of comfort. A useful checklist in client preparation includes:

- Does the client need to visit the toilet prior to treatment? Failure to do so may cause discomfort and distraction.
- How much fluid have they drunk today? Offer a glass of water to help to cleanse and rehydrate the systems prior to treatment. Very few people drink enough water and as a result suffer the effects associated with varying levels of dehydration including discomfort.
- Have they eaten today? Offer a client who has not eaten for over five hours a couple of dry, plain biscuits. Lack of food results in physical and psychological weakness, making the whole body more vulnerable and uncomfortable as a result.
- Ask the client to remove any tight, restrictive clothing or jewellery that may cause discomfort affecting blood and energy flow to the area.
- Check temperature with the client and adjust the covering of their body with towels, blankets or a duvet accordingly.
- Check general comfort and put in place additional support (rolled-up towels, pillows) as required.

Observation of client body language will help to determine their level of comfort. It is usual for a client, especially if they have not had a treatment before, to be quite guarded at the start of the treatment and they may fold their arms in front of them. Whilst it makes sense to ask them to lay their arms by their side a more gentle approach may be to monitor their responses to the relaxation techniques used and adapt them in terms of timing and pressure until the client becomes naturally more relaxed and open to treatment.

Knowledge review

1   What is the main priority of the reflexology treatment?

2   What response does stress initiate in the body?

3   Name the special senses responsible for picking up stress.

4   Name the three hormones that are released in response to stress.

5   What does the abbreviation GAS stand for?

6   What are the three stages associated with GAS?

7   Name three effects of long-term unsafe stress.

8   Explain the terms direct and indirect reflexes.

9   Give an example of a cross-reflex.

10   What products may be used during treatment and why?

13

Anatomy and physiology overview

The natural progression from consultation to treatment commences once the initial questions have been asked and the relevant paper work completed (see Part 3 for consultation forms), the area to be treated has been isolated and examined and relaxation movements applied. The commercial timing of the whole treatment inclusive of the consultation is generally approximately one-and-a-quarter hours for a new client, with subsequent treatments taking in the region of 45 minutes to an hour.

The treatment itself encompasses all of the body systems and organs and this may be completed generally by working over each foot, hand or ear in turn or specifically by working the reflex points for each system on both feet, hands or ears simultaneously.

It is common practice to make use of a treatment plan to record the findings associated with the treatment of each reflex point.

 Angel advice

Further reference should be made to anatomy and physiology books e.g. *An Holistic Guide to Anatomy and Physiology*.

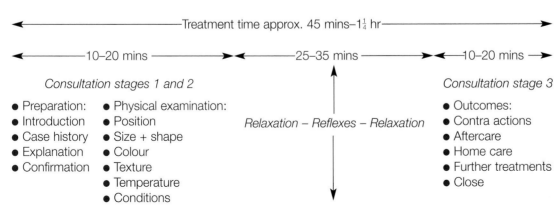

Treatment time line

REFLEXOLOGY TREATMENT CARD

Name .... Date ....

Relaxation   [   ]   Comments ....

Zones – systemic systems   ....

                [   ]   ....

Skeletal/Muscular systems

R Cranium	L Cranium	R Face	L Face
R Neck	L Neck	R top & sides	L top & sides

Spine – Cervical

R1	L1	R2	L2	R3	L3	R4	L4	R5	L5	R6	L6	R7	L7

Spine – Thoracic

R1	L1	R2	L2	R3	L3	R4	L4	R5	L5	R6	L6
R7	L7	R8	L8	R9	L9	R10	L10	R11	L11	R12	L12

Spine – Lumbar

R1	L1	R2	L2	R3	L3	R4	L4	R5	L5

R Sacrum	L Sacrum	R Coccyx	L Coccyx	R Sciatic	L Sciatic
R Thorax	L Thorax				

Joints

R Shoulder	L Shoulder	R Elbow	L Elbow	R Wrist	L Wrist
R Hip	L Hip	R Knee	L Knee	R Ankle	L Ankle

Respiratory system

R Throat	L Throat	R Ear	L Ear	
R Eust Tube	L Eust Tube	R Eye	L Eye	
R Sinus	L Sinus	R Jaw	L Jaw	
R Trachea	L Trachea	R Lung	L Lung	Solar Plexus

Digestive system

R Oes	L Oes	Stomach	Pancreas	Duodenum
Spleen	Liver	Gall Bladder	Small Intest	Appendix
Illeocaecal	Asc Colon	Hepatic Fl	Trans Colon	Splenic Fl
Desc Colon	Sig Colon	Anus		

Genito-Urinary system

R Ov/Test	L Ov/Test	R Fall/VasDef	L Fall/VasDef	
R Uterus/Pros	L Uterus/Pros			
R Kidney	L Kidney	R Ureter	L Ureter	Bladder

Endocrine system

R Pituitary	L Pituitary	R Pineal	L Pineal	
R Thyroid	L Thyroid	R Parathyroid	L Parathyroid	
R Thymus	L Thymus	R Adrenal	L Adrenal	

Lymphatic system

R Breast	L Breast	R Groin	L Groin	
R Joints	L Joints	R Spine	L Spine	

Relaxation   [   ]   Breathing Exercises

L = left, R = right

To appreciate this, it is vital that the reflexology practitioner has a working knowledge of anatomy and physiology.

Systems of the body

A new organism is formed via the reproductive systems of a male and female through the process of **meiosis**, whereby fusion of a sperm from the male with an **ovum** (egg) from the female takes place. The creation of this organism into a human being occurs through the process of **mitosis** whereby cells divide and specialise, forming individual organs and systems, eventually developing into a fully formed and functional body, mind and spirit.

In order to sustain life the human body is required to make use of vital resources in the form of **air**, **water** and **food**. The utilisation of these resources takes place through the functioning of the body systems:

- Air is breathed into the body through the **respiratory system** where oxygen, the gas vital for life is absorbed. As a result of the body using oxygen, carbon dioxide is formed and this is released from the body when breathing out.

- Water is taken into the body through the **digestive system**, where this vital nutrient for life is absorbed. Any excess water is collected by the body and excreted via the **urinary system** in the form of urine.

- Food is also taken into the body through the **digestive system**, where the vital nutrients for life are broken down and absorbed. As a result of this process waste products are generated and released from the body via the same system.

Air, water and food are transported around the body by means of the **circulatory systems**, with the **blood circulation** forming a continuous network of tubes (arteries and veins) supplying every living cell with the means for survival and the **lymphatic circulation** forming a one-way system helping to collect up the waste products associated with this interaction for removal from the body.

This process is controlled by the **central nervous system** (CNS) (the brain and spinal cord) which is able to coordinate the activity in all parts of the body through the **peripheral nervous system** (PNS) (sensory and motor nerves) affecting the voluntary movements associated with the **muscular** and **skeletal systems** and the **autonomic nervous system** (ANS) (sympathetic and parasympathetic systems) affecting the involuntary muscular activity associated with body functions such as digestion. The nervous system in turn links with the **endocrine system** which activates the release of hormones into the bloodstream. **Hormones** have an additional controlling action on the development of the body through the cycles of life e.g. waking and sleeping, puberty, pregnancy and menopause.

The body as a whole relies on a combination of organs from related systems to form the **immune system**, which in turn protects the body against external and internal attack.

In addition to the nutrients vital for life in the form of air, water and food, the body also relies on the external energy that it receives from the world around it. Energy is generated from the sun and earth and between living beings. This energy is absorbed into the body through the **integumentary system** (skin, hair and nails) as well as through the special senses (ears, eyes, nose and tongue) interpreted via the nervous system and acted upon via the relevant body systems.

By working in harmony together, the body systems are able to create the ideal environment for life, providing the means for all vital functions to take place i.e. **respiration, metabolism, immunity, sensation, movement, excretion** and **reproduction**:

- Respiration – gaseous interchange between the cells of the body and the external environment.
- Metabolism – the physical and chemical processes of the body.
- Immunity – the body's resistance to disease.
- Sensation – the ability to respond to a stimulus by interpreting it as a physical, psychological or spiritual feeling.
- Movement – the voluntary action of skeletal muscles and the involuntary action of cardiac and visceral muscles in coordinating movement of the body.
- Excretion – the removal of waste products from the cells.
- Reproduction – the fusion of the sperm and the ova for the survival of the species.

Just as each individual body system relies on this interaction for its survival, so do individual cells of the body, therefore we cannot be well unless the whole is well.

Reflexology supports this theory in two ways:

1. By working *generally* over the whole of the feet, hands and/or ears the body is benefiting from an overall stimulation of all of its parts.
2. By isolating each organ and body system on the feet, hands and/or ears in turn, each body part is benefiting *specifically* i.e. by adapting the pressure and length of time spent on each part the benefits can be specifically stimulating or soothing depending on its needs.

Treatment of the body systems with reflexology

The systemic body systems – i.e. those which pertain to or affect the body as a whole – can be treated by working generally. Therefore by working over the whole of the feet, hands or ears the treatment will affect the following systems:

- Nervous system

- Circulatory systems

- Integumentary system

- Immune system

The other systems of the body are more specific in their positions and their functions and so can be more easily accessed for specific treatment. Some systems may be linked for treatment and include:

- Skeletal/muscular systems

- Respiratory system

- Digestive system

- Genito-urinary system

- Endocrine system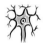

- Lymphatic system

These systems are highlighted for treatment in Chapters 14–19.

To understand how a general treatment can be of benefit to the systemic systems of the body it is useful to have a working knowledge of their basic **structure and function, consultation considerations** and **common conditions** affecting their well-being.

Structure and function

Nervous system

The nervous system controls the body with electrical impulses, allowing it to detect external and internal changes and to make use of the information received to form a response. It forms vital links with all of the systems of the body, providing them with the ability to feel and respond. Nerve cells called **neurons** facilitate this action:

- Sensory neurons carry impulses to the brain.
- Motor neurons carry impulses away from the brain.

The brain and spinal cord coordinate these impulses through the peripheral nervous system, which consists of:

- 12 pairs of cranial nerves servicing the face and neck and responsible for our sense of smell, sight, taste, balance and hearing as well as such functions as breathing, eating speaking and feeling.
- 31 pairs of spinal nerves servicing the rest of the body with functions associated with feeling and movement of the corresponding areas of the body.

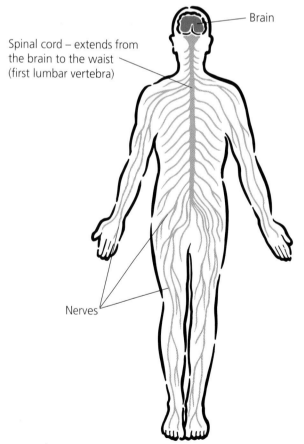

Brain

Spinal cord – extends from the brain to the waist (first lumbar vertebra)

Nerves

The nervous system

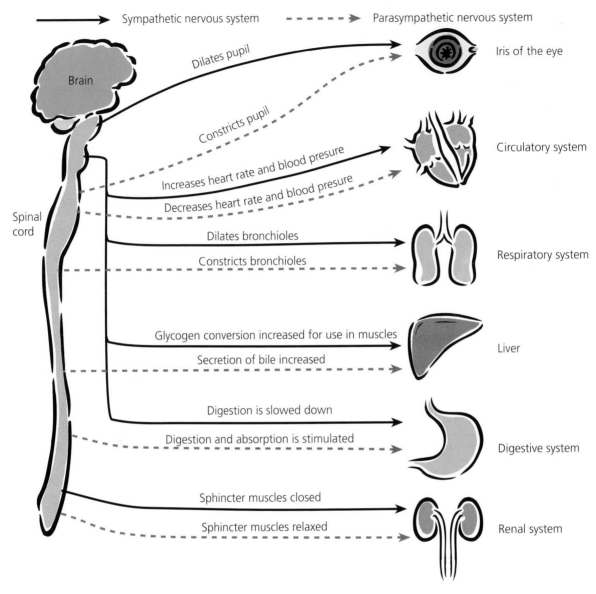

The autonomic nervous system

The autonomic nervous systems controls the body further by responding to the effects of stress by:

- The sympathetic system preparing the body for activity.
- The parasympathetic system preparing the body for rest.

Circulatory system

The circulatory system consists of two complementary systems, blood and lymphatic circulation, which work together in providing the whole of the body with a transportation system. The blood circulation is a two-way system that:

- Transports the vital resources such as oxygen, water and food *to* every cell of the body via arteries, arterioles and capillaries.

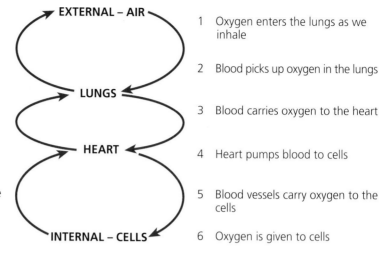

12 Carbon dioxide leaves the lungs as we exhale

11 Blood gives carbon dioxide to the lungs

10 Blood carries carbon dioxide to the lungs

9 Heart pumps blood to the lungs

8 Blood vessels carry carbon dioxide to the heart

7 Cells give carbon dioxide to the blood

EXTERNAL – AIR

LUNGS

HEART

INTERNAL – CELLS

1 Oxygen enters the lungs as we inhale

2 Blood picks up oxygen in the lungs

3 Blood carries oxygen to the heart

4 Heart pumps blood to cells

5 Blood vessels carry oxygen to the cells

6 Oxygen is given to cells

The blood circulatory system

- Transports unwanted substances such as carbon dioxide and waste products *away* from every cell via capillaries, venules and veins to be released out of the body.

The lymphatic circulation is a one-way system which supports the blood circulation (see Chapter 19).

The heart forms the central part of the circulatory system, coordinating the flow of oxygenated blood *from* the lungs and deoxygenated blood *to* the lungs via:

- Pulmonory circulation between the heart and lungs.
- Systemic circulation between the heart and the cells.
- Portal circulation between the heart and the digestive system.
- Coronary circulation between the heart and its own tissues.

Integumentary system

The integumentary system consists of the skin, hair and nails providing the whole body with a waterproof protective outer covering that is resilient, flexible and contributes to our unique personal appearance. The skin forms three distinct layers:

1. The inner most layer or **hypodermis** consisting of connective tissue forming an insulating layer for the storage of fat cells.
2. The **dermis** lies directly above the hypodermis and forms the true skin containing the hair follicles, sweat and sebaceous glands and arrector pili muscles together with collagen, elastin and reticulin fibres and a rich blood and nerve supply.
3. The **epidermis** forms the upper most layer of skin and is made up of five layers that contribute to the protective function and external appearance of the skin and nails.

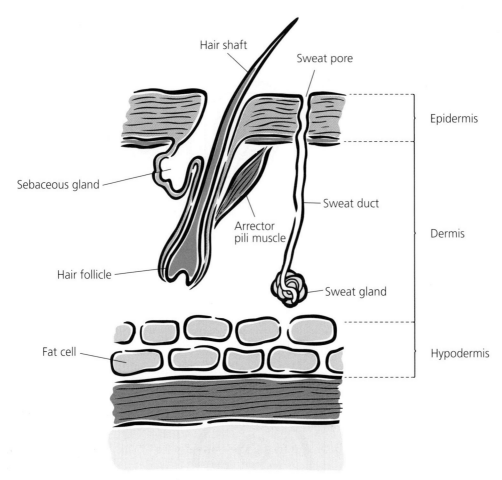

The structure of the skin

Immune system

The immune system comprises of aspects of each body system in the fight for survival:

- Cells – leucocytes or white blood cells defend the body against attack from bacteria, viruses etc.

- Tissue – epithelial tissue forms the linings or coverings of many organs and vessels and forms the first line of defence against attack e.g. skin.

- Glands – comprised of lymphatic tissue to help to filter unwanted substances from the body e.g. lymph nodes, adenoids, tonsils, appendix, thymus gland etc.

- Organs – most organs are involved with some form of detoxification, filtration and/or elimination of waste from the body e.g. the liver detoxifies the blood ridding it of drugs and alcohol, the kidneys filter waste from the blood, the skin eliminates small amounts of waste in the form of sweat etc.

- Systems – all systems of the body are involved in the body's defence mechanisms against internal and external attack and will support each other in the fight for survival.

System sorter

CELLS

Nervous system

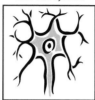

Specialist cells known as neurons and neuroglia form nervous tissue. Their function of sensitivity enables the body to respond to external and internal stimuli. Reflexology helps to stimulate nerve responses, making the system more efficient and effective.

Circulatory system

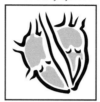

Blood cells form fluid connective tissue. They are able to move around the body within tubes (arteries and veins) transporting substances to and from all of the other cells of the body for growth, repair and maintenance. Reflexology stimulates blood flow, speeding up its transportation functions.

Integumentary system

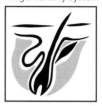

The cells of the surface of the skin, hair and nails form stratified keratinised epithelial tissue. This means that they are formed in layers, are hard and dry and contain the protein keratin, thus contributing to the protection of the body as a whole. Skin cells are constantly being renewed and reflexology stimulates this process.

Skeletal/muscular systems

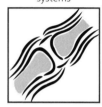

Specialised cells form the dense tissue associated with bones and the different types of muscular tissue needed for voluntary and involuntary movement of the body as a whole. Reflexology helps to stimulate all forms of movement, making the body perform more effectively as a whole.

Immune system

The body protects itself generally by providing non-specific defence through organs such as the skin and the linings of the nose and digestive tracts and functions such as fever and inflammation. The body is also able to target specific disease-causing agents known as pathogens by providing specific defence or immunity. Reflexology helps to activate these mechanisms.

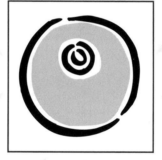

The respiratory tracts – nose, throat, windpipe – that lead into the lungs contain a lining that is ciliated. This means there is a covering of tiny hairs (cilia) which trap unwanted particles preventing them from entering the body. Reflexology helps to relax the body which in turn relaxes the airways, allowing improved breathing.

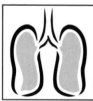

Respiratory system

The lining of the bladder is formed from transitional epithelial tissue which is contractible, allowing the bladder to expand when full of urine and deflate when empty. Reflexology stimulates activity in all areas of the genito-urinary system, helping related organs to work together harmoniously.

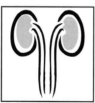

Genito-urinary system

Endocrine glands are formed from epithelial tissue and contain cells which are able to secrete a hormone (a chemical messenger) directly into the blood stream. The blood transports hormones to target cells which pick up the associated message and act accordingly. Reflexology helps to balance the secretion of hormones, aiding in homeostasis.

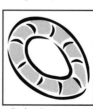

Endocrine system

Lymphatic tissue is semi-solid tissue which contains specialist cells that help to control disease by engulfing bacteria. It forms nodes, glands and ducts. Lymph is a liquid similar to blood which helps to pick up cellular waste along with blood. Reflexology stimulates lymphatic activity, helping to rid the body of harmful waste and fight disease.

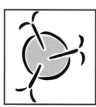

Lymphatic system

The lining of the digestive tract is made up of goblet cells that are responsible for the secretion of mucus. This mucus helps the flow of nutrients and waste through the system. Reflexology stimulates the action within the digestive system, allowing more effective absorption of nutrients and more efficient removal of waste.

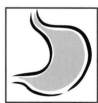

Digestive system

Consultation considerations

As discussed in Part Three, it is important to take a detailed case history in order to ascertain the general state of well-being of the body as a whole. Disharmony in any one of the systemic systems will have far-reaching effects on the rest of the body because of their generic links and considerations should include:

Oral

Questions relating to levels of sensitivity, temperature, frequency and type of skin problems and minor ailments will determine the general state of these systems and provide a basis for many related problems e.g.

- Lack of sensation indicates problems with the cranial or spinal nerves e.g. lack of skin sensitivity, eye strain, loss of the sense of smell etc.
- If the person is always cold, circulation will be poor and body systems will suffer.
- Increased body temperature may be caused by stress to the systems.
- Skin problems may be caused by localised problems and/or systemic problems.
- Minor ailments signify an imbalance in the immune functions of the body.

Visual

First impressions provide us with a means to determine the well-being of these systemic systems e.g.

- A thick, full head of hair denotes a good and healthy circulation.
- A glow to the skin tells us that these systems are working in harmony together.
- Clear, bright eyes indicate general good health.

Aural

The consultation is about so much more than just asking a set of questions and hearing the answers. Listening to the words said and the words left unsaid during periods of silence help to determine the true meaning of the answers given. Often descriptive statements can help to create greater understanding e.g. 'it made my blood boil' or 'it made the hairs on the back of my neck stand on end' tell us more about the emotional state of a person than that of their blood circulation, integumentary or nervous systems!

Angel advice

Often, hours after the treatment I suddenly realise the meaning of something a client has said or done that was not at all obvious to me during the consultation or indeed the treatment. It is important to have time for reflection, which in turn brings greater insight and understanding.

Olfactory

The sense of smell is an underused skill that can contribute greatly to the effectiveness of the consultation. The use of all of our senses helps to build a total picture of a person and no one skill should be in any way underestimated, even though it may at first appear irrelevant. It is useful to pick up on any unusual odour and use a process of elimination to determine its possible cause which may be external – the use of perfumes etc. – and/or internal – e.g. the malfunction of a systemic or localised body part or system.

Perceptive

The power of perception will help to alert the practitioner to the needs of each client, helping to build awareness and make a route for adaptation of treatment. The systemic systems affect every aspect of the human body and as such provide an insight that is difficult to ignore. It is useful to be aware of the fact that so much information may be conflicting and confusing with the potential to cause information overload! Information should be picked up over a period of time, but also, time should be provided to make sense of the information so that it can be put to good use in the future.

Tactile

The feel of the part of body being touched will help to determine the state of well-being associated with it:

- The first point of any contact is with the integumentary system and the overall feel of the skin, hair and nails will provide a vital insight into the overall state of the body, e.g. a dry skin may indicate dryness in the body as a whole, alerting the practitioner to a person's fluid intake.
- Blood flow to the area may be felt in the temperature of the skin, with a cold skin indicating that circulation may be poor.
- Imbalanced immunity and nervous function may be felt by extremes e.g. pain or lack of any sensation.

Care should be taken to adapt the pressure of touch to meet the needs of the area being treated and the person being treated.

Contraindication considerations

Any major conditions, disorders or illnesses affecting these systems should be given careful consideration before the treatment takes place e.g.

- Infectious diseases may result in cross-infection.
- Conditions requiring surgery and/or recent surgery may be adversely affected by treatment, possibly impeding healing.

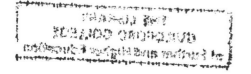

- Conditions affecting the circulatory system may be stimulated due to the effects of massage e.g. varicose veins, thrombosis, heart conditions etc.
- Early stages of pregnancy for fear of miscarriage.
- Undiagnosed swellings and/or lumps may be adversely stimulated.
- Some medications may be affected by the cleansing reaction of the treatment, making them less effective.

Reflexology is viewed as a complementary treatment and as such may be used to enhance any treatment provided by the medical profession. Professional ethics should be observed when dealing with a client who is undergoing medical treatment, and advice should be sought from their specialist as to the suitability of the reflexology treatment. This is not to say that someone suffering with any of these conditions is necessarily contraindicated to treatment, just that special care should be taken to ensure that the treatment remains complementary and above all safe.

Angel advice

The medical world is still divided in their knowledge and belief of reflexology. Time, education and patience are gradually bringing the two elements of health care together.

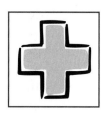

Common conditions

When conducting a consultation in preparation for a reflexology treatment, careful consideration needs to be given to conditions relating to each of the systemic body systems as well as those which affect the other individual systems. Such conditions do not occur in isolation. Working over the entire feet, hands or ears will have a beneficial effect on all the conditions affecting the systemic systems.

Common conditions of the nervous system

- ALZHEIMER'S DISEASE – a gradual shrinking of the brain where the nerve fibres become tangled, resulting in a progressive decline in mental activities.
- BELL'S PALSY – inflammation of the facial nerve resulting in sudden paralysis causing one side of the face to drop. Complete recovery usually occurs within a few weeks.
- CEREBRAL PALSY – a permanent disorder of the brain affecting the control of muscles. Muscles have reduced control and go into spasms.
- CLUSTER HEADACHE – severe headache that starts three to four hours after falling asleep, recurs nightly for weeks or months and then disappears for years. More common in men than in women.
- DELERIUM TREMENS (dt's) – confusion, hallucinations and trembling associated with the withdrawal symptoms which occur when an alcoholic stops drinking.
- DEMENTIA – gradual death of brain cells through normal ageing. Memory loss, confusion and changes in behaviour may result.

- EPILEPSY – temporary loss of consciousness. It is known as petit mal when loss of consciousness is for a few seconds, and grand mal when unconsciousness is accompanied by convulsions.
- MENINGITIS – a severe infection of the membrane surrounding the brain and spinal cord.
- MIGRAINE – recurrent severe headache with additional symptoms including flashing lights before the eyes together with a dislike of bright lights. Nausea and vomiting may also occur.
- MOTOR NEURON DISEASE – a condition which affects the motor neurons, causing progressive weakness in the muscles.
- MULTIPLE SCLEROSIS (MS) – degeneration of the nervous tissue in the central nervous tissue. This disease starts in adults between the ages of 20–50 and affects the parts of the body controlled by those sections of damaged nervous tissue including vision, speech, movement etc.
- NEURALGIA – pressure on a nerve caused by irritation. Pain may be felt along the length of the nerve as well as at the point of pressure.
- NEURITIS – inflammation of nerves resulting in muscle weakness and loss of skin sensitivity.
- NEUROSIS – excessive feelings of anxiety, depression and/or phobia.
- NOCTURNAL MYOCLONUS – a sudden jerking of muscles as a person is drifting off to sleep, causing momentary panic. If this occurs frequently it can interfere with sleep.
- PARKINSON'S DISEASE – muscular stiffness and tremors develop as the parts of the base of the brain degenerate leading to a deficiency of dopamine which aids the transmission of nerve impulses.
- SCIATICA – abnormal pressure on any part of the length of the sciatic nerve, which extends down the legs from the lower back, resulting in pain.
- SPINA BIFIDA – a condition that is present at birth. Spinal nerves are affected due to malformation of bones and tissue surrounding the spine resulting in mental and/or physical handicap.
- STRESS – prolonged, unsafe stress places pressure on all aspects of the nervous system resulting in physical and psychological symptoms e.g. headaches and strong emotions.
- STROKE – a sudden loss of function on one side of the body caused by an interruption of the blood supply to part of the brain.
- TENSION HEADACHE – pain resulting from overworked muscles of the scalp, face and neck often associated with excessive concentration.
- VERTIGO – feeling of dizziness when standing still.

Common conditions of the circulatory system

Fascinating Fact

Beta blockers are drugs used to decrease the workload of the heart.

- ANAEMIA – a decrease in the production of red blood cells and/or haemoglobin. This may be caused by excessive blood loss reducing the amount of red blood cells in the body, lack of iron affecting the haemoglobin function or dysfunction in the bone marrow resulting in loss of production of new blood cells.
- ANEURYSM – localised swelling of an artery which can develop if the artery is diseased or weakened, especially if blood pressure is high.
- ANGINA – reduction of blood flow to the heart, usually brought on by excessive exertion.
- ARRHYTHMIA – irregular heartbeat causing quickening of the heart on inspiration and slowing on expiration.
- ARTERIAL THROMBOSIS – clotting of blood in an artery obstructing normal blood flow.
- ARTERIOSCLEROSIS – the walls of the arteries lose their elasticity and harden. This has the effect of raising the blood pressure.
- ARTERITIS – inflammation of an artery, often associated with rheumatoid arthritis.
- ATHEROSCLEROSIS – a narrowing of the arteries caused by a build up of fats including cholesterol.
- CORONARY THROMBOSIS – a common cause of heart attacks where an artery supplying the heart is obstructed.
- HYPERTENSION – high blood pressure.
- HYPOTENSION – low blood pressure.
- STRESS – prolonged, unsafe stress puts strain on the heart and blood vessels.
- THROMBO PHLEBITIS – inflammation of the length of a vein, usually occurring in the legs.
- VARICOSE VEINS – ineffective valves in veins cause the blood to collect in the veins instead of returning to the heart. This results in veins becoming distended and painful.

Common conditions of the integumentary system

- ACNE – there are two types of acne: acne rosacea and acne vulgaris. Acne rosacea results in redness of the nose and cheeks caused by dilation of capillaries. Acne vulgaris results in blocked and sometimes infected sebaceous glands commonly affecting the face, neck, back and chest.
- ALLERGIES – sensitivity causing the skin to react adversely by becoming red, hot and itchy. An allergy is the response to the alarm reaction and forms a part of the body's defence mechanism, alerting the body to potential attack from foreign bodies.

- ALOPECIA – baldness caused by hair follicles being unable to produce new hairs. This may be in specific areas – known as alopecia areata – or total hair loss from the scalp – known as alopecia totalis. Total loss of hair from the whole of the body is known as alopecia universalis.
- ASTEATOSIS – underactive sebaceous glands causing excessively dry, scaly and often itchy skin.
- CREEPING CELLULITIS – spreading inflammation of the skin. Skin is hot to touch, tender and shiny.
- CHILBLAINS – painful red, blue or purple areas of skin found on the toes and fingers as a result of poor circulation.
- BRUISE – discolouration in or below the skin tissue resulting from an injury. Blood leaks from damaged blood vessels into the surrounding tissue.
- ECZEMA/DERMATITIS – inflammation of the skin. Eczema starts with redness due to dilated blood vessels, fluid accumulates in the skin causing swelling, itching and blisters. Weeping skin develops and may become infected. It eventually dries to form scabs and crusts.
- FUNGAL INFECTIONS – ringworm including tinea corporis affecting the skin, tinea pedis affecting the feet and onychmycosis affecting the nails. Fungal infections are highly contagious.
- HYPERIDROSIS – excessive sweating affecting areas such as the hands, feet and underarms.
- PSORIASIS – a recurring scaly eruption of the skin. Red patches develop, covered by a scale which may be itchy.
- VIRAL INFECTIONS – including herpes simplex affecting the skin surrounding the mouth, herpes zoster or shingles affecting the body. Warts and veruccas are also caused by viral infection. Viral infections are highly contagious.

Fascinating Fact

A treatment for severe hyperidrosis is injecting of Botox, which causes a semi-permanent paralysis of the sweat glands.

Common conditions of the immune system

- AIDS – Acquired Immune Deficiency Syndrome caused by the HIV Human Immune Deficiency virus. The T-lymphocytes are attacked making the immune system incapable of functioning effectively.
- MYALGIC ENCEPHALITIS (ME) – also referred to as post-viral fatigue and resembles the symptoms that follow many viral infections including muscle pain, fatigue, exhaustion, depression etc. Symptoms may last for several months and even years.
- STRESS – any factor that exerts a negative effect on the body, which if allowed to continue results in gradual degeneration of body systems and associated functions. The effects of prolonged negative stress may be seen in the condition of the hair, skin and nails.

Treatment tracker

CELLS

Visualisation

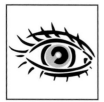

Hands

Feet

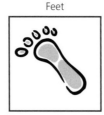

Ears

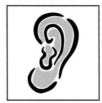

Affirmation

Visualisation provides a means of exerting mind over matter. In effect it is a way of guiding the body through a course of action, which at best can have a therapeutic positive effect with nice thoughts and at worst a very detrimental negative effect with not so nice thoughts! In turn, visualisations have a knock-on effect on stress levels as we see events occurring in our mind's eye. Using visualisation to guide your body to a better place gives a sense of freedom that is within easy grasp of anyone opening their mind to endless possibilities as we explore the times and places which evoke positive thoughts and feelings. To start the practice of visualisation, it is useful to pick a time and/or place in your life, whether real or imaginary, that fills you with good feelings. The good feelings that these images evoke naturally counteract bad feelings, thus instilling the body with a greater sense of balance. Visualisation appeals to left-brain dominant types.

The hands as a whole are representational of the systemic systems i.e. nervous, circulatory, integumentary and immune. Specific reflex points include the heart, which is located predominantly on the left hand in the upper section of the palm, the brain, which is located in the tip of the thumb and the spinal cord, which is located along the medial edge of the hands.

Like the hands, the feet are also representational of the systemic systems as a whole. The specific reflex point of the heart is located predominantly on the left foot in the upper section of the sole. The brain reflex point is found in the tip of the big toe and the spinal cord reflex is located along the medial edge of the feet.

As with the hands and feet, the systemic systems are represented in the whole of the ear with the heart reflex located in the lower concha, the brain in the upper section of the ear lobe and the spinal cord along the base of the antihelix. The reflex points of the ear are much smaller than those of the hands and feet, but working generally over the systemic systems will have the same effect.

Affirmations make use of the spoken word either as an imagined sound or one actually spoken out loud. We sometimes hear people refer to the fact that they gave themselves 'a good talking to' – this forms the basis of the use of affirmations. It may be in the form of a positive word or phrase that sums up a person's intent e.g. 'I will finish writing this book/essay/case study etc. because I appreciate having the opportunity to do so'. Sometimes in everyday life the intent gets lost, as we try to cope with the stresses and strains of completing the task along with everything else that life throws our way. Instead of focusing on the negative, the use of affirmations enables us to take a positive focal point along.

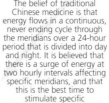

The belief of traditional Chinese medicine is that energy flows in a continuous, never ending cycle through the meridians over a 24-hour period that is divided into day and night. It is believed that there is a surge of energy at two hourly intervals affecting specific meridians, and that this is the best time to stimulate specific organs/systems within each meridian – when their energy is said to be 'full'.

It is also believed that for every two hour surge of energy there is an opposing two hour period of sedation of energy. This concept has the potential to have an effect on a reflexology treatment e.g. sometimes an organ or a system may appear to 'come up' simply because of this natural energy surge. It is therefore useful to be aware of the position of the meridians and the timing of the natural energy movement when treating clients at different times of the day.

Colour can be introduced in a variety of ways and can form a useful part of any aftercare procedures. The systemic systems of the body are associated predominantly with the colours red and yellow:

- Red stimulates circulation and promotes body heat and adrenalin production. It is useful for times when the body is feeling emotionally and physically low.
- Yellow is at the centre of the whole of the nervous system (the brain and spinal cord) and of the autonomic nervous system (the solar plexus). It is associated with the power of self-control and has a controlling effect on the automatic functions of the body e.g. breathing, digestion, elimination etc.

The systemic systems are associated with all seven chakras as their combined energies affect the whole of the body and are associated with survival, clairsentience, (the perception of other people's emotions), energy, love, communication, clairvoyance and intuition. In addition to the seven main chakras, there are also two secondary groups of chakras that are found in the feet and hands. The feet chakras are located on the soles of the feet and help to maintain a person's connection with the earth. The hand chakras are located on the palms of the hands and are the centre of creative energy. The energy generated from the hand chakras is associated with hands-on healing.

The systemic systems are represented in all five longitudinal zones and all three transverse zones. The longitudinal zones run from each finger and toe; the transverse zones run between the shoulder and diaphragm line, the diaphragm and waistline and the waistline and pelvic line. The body can be mapped out in the zones making the pinpointing of specific reflexes easier. By working the length and breadth of the zones we can be sure of treating the systemic systems, which will have an indirect effect on the rest of the body.

- The heart meridian starts in the underarm and ends at the back of the little finger and is naturally stimulated between 11 a.m.–1 p.m. and is naturally sedated between 11 p.m. and 1 a.m.
- The pericardium meridian starts from the chest and descends down the arm to the back of the middle finger and is naturally stimulated between 7 p.m.–9 p.m. and naturally sedated between 7 a.m.–9 a.m.

The use of sound can also be introduced into the treatment as well as form a useful addition to any aftercare advice given. The notes C and F are predominantly associated with the nervous system.

- C affects the circulation and music with a set, even beat is useful in regulating the flow of blood around the body.
- F affects all aspects of the nervous system and all forms of classical music provide suitable stimulation.

The use of sound appeals to right-brain dominant types.

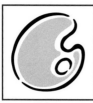

Colour

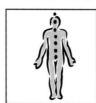

Chakras

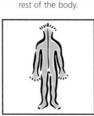

Zones

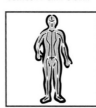

Meridians

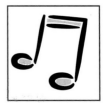

Sound

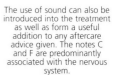

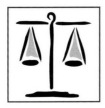

Holistic harmony

There is nothing about the human body that works in isolation. Every cell, tissue, gland, organ and system is reliant on the interaction of other cells, tissues, glands, organs and systems for their state of well-being. Homeostasis can only be maintained if there is internal harmony.

The saying 'what goes around, comes around' is very apt in describing the condition of the human body. The way in which the body is treated throughout life will offer repercussions in future well-being. With this in mind, thought should be given to the level of responsibility we each have for the care of our own bodies. This care forms a vital part of the continuation of a reflexology treatment. Information relating to the quality, quantity and effects on the body, mind and spirit of **air**, **water**, **nutrition**, **rest**, **activity**, **age**, **awareness** and **special care** forms a part of the aftercare advice given at the end of each reflexology treatment.

Air

The air we breathe contains the main nutrient vital for life – oxygen. A good supply of oxygen is needed to maintain the functions of the systemic systems:

- Approximately 2,000 litres of blood pass through the brain every day, allowing the absorption of about 60 litres of oxygen. Unlike other cells, the body cannot generally replace nerve cells so their need for oxygen is paramount to prevent deterioration.

- Red blood cells contain haemoglobin which is responsible for the transportation of oxygen to the cells of the body. Certain gases present in the air, e.g. carbon monoxide, affect the haemoglobin making the transportation of oxygen difficult.

- Any toxins from the environment are absorbed into the body through the integumentary system, breaking down the protective acid mantle resulting in skin, hair and nails that are more vulnerable and prone to problems.

- The quality of air also has a direct effect on the immune functions of the body. Impure air breathed into the body stimulates immunity in order to prevent the body from coming under attack by foreign bodies that may be present in the air. This may have a long-term debilitating effect on the immune functions, e.g. the damaging effect of one cigarette may be counteracted by the stimulation of blood cells in response to smoking. However, the long-term effects of smoking push the limits of the body, resulting in possible illness.

Water

The body is made up of a large percentage of water (roughly 75 per cent) which is present in each of the systemic body systems.

- Intracellular fluid – makes up the water found in the cells.
- Extracellular fluid – makes up the water found in body fluids e.g. blood, mucus etc.

Nervous tissue, blood, skin, hair, nails and lymphatic tissue all rely on water for the maintenance of their functions.

- The brain is made up of 75 per cent water and water is needed by neurons to facilitate the action of electrical impulses through the nerve fibres.
- Approximately 90 per cent of blood plasma is water in which chemical substances are dissolved or suspended.
- Not only is water contained in the layers of the skin, hair and nails, but it also forms the sweat and sebum secreted from the sudoriferous and sebaceous glands.
- Immune functions rely on there being adequate amounts of water available within the body.

Eating and drinking provides the body with most of the water needed and this is known as performed water. Metabolic water refers to that which is produced through catabolism (cellular function).

The body requires in the region of one-and-a-half litres of performed water to prevent dehydration. Dehydration starts to occur when the body loses more water than it takes in. Varying levels of dehydration are now thought to contribute to the causes of many common conditions including headaches, morning sickness, skin problems, rheumatoid pain, anginal pain etc.

Reflexology can help to identify levels of dehydration through treatment and encourage and/or reinforce the introduction of more good fluid, i.e. water and less bad fluid, i.e. caffeine and alcohol.

Nutrition

In addition to air and water, the body relies on the nutrients gained from the foods we eat to maintain its functions. Digested food is absorbed into the bloodstream and transported around the body for use by every living cell.

Nutrients vital for maintaining homeostasis within the systemic body systems also contribute to levels of balance within the body as a whole and include:

- **Proteins** – needed by the body for growth and repair.
- **Carbohydrates** – used by the body in the production of energy.
- **Fats** – provide the body with an additional source of fuel.
- **Minerals** and **vitamins** – essential for all processes within the body.

A balanced diet is needed to ensure that the systems of the body maintain balanced levels of activity (see Chapter 16 – the digestive system for more details).

Reflexology helps to encourage better nutrition by creating awareness through treatment and building understanding through aftercare.

Rest

All body systems need periods of rest to allow the body to counteract the actions involved in periods of activity. As with all things, the body craves balance. Rest may be put into two categories – relaxation and sleep.

- Relaxation offers the body a period of rest during which time there is a lessening of physical and psychological tension.
- Sleep offers the body a period of rest during which voluntary action and consciousness are either in partial or complete abeyance.

Times of rest vary with age, activity, lifestyle and stress levels, with babies needing more sleep (an average of 16 hours per day) than the elderly (an average of 5 hours per day).

Without adequate periods of resting time the systemic body systems become tired and demonstrate the following symptoms:

- Nerve responses become slower, concentration times lessen and the brain feels muddled and overloaded.
- Sensory organs e.g. the eyes may become strained with tiredness affecting vision etc.
- Venous blood flow may be impeded as it fights against the pull of gravity back to the heart.
- The skin, hair and nails become dull and lifeless with the finer skin around the eyes developing dark shadows.
- Extreme tiredness often results in low immunity as the protective functions of the body become affected.

Reflexology encourages periods of rest through relaxation and, as a result of the treatment, periods of rest through sleep are also improved.

Activity

In the same way that the body and its systems need periods of rest, they also need periods of activity in order to maintain homeostasis. It is true to say that 'if you don't use it, you'll lose it' as body functions diminish through lack of use.

- The nervous system relies on mental and physical activity to keep it healthy.
- Venous blood flow relies on the action of skeletal muscles for the flow of blood back to the heart.
- The integumentary system relies on physical activity to stimulate blood flow for the continuous renewal of skin, hair and nail cells.

Angel advice

Think about the way in which we can exert mental activity to activate the mind over matter effect. Many people rely on this positive effect as an additional aid in the healing of the body.

- The immune system relies on physical and psychological activity to stimulate the actions of its structures in the fight against disease.

Reflexology provides a means to activate the systemic systems of the body through the application of massage and the use of varying depths of pressure.

Age

Ageing is associated with the progressive failure of the body systems to maintain homeostasis. The majority of cells within the body are able to reproduce themselves by mitosis e.g. skin cells. Research is showing that certain cells have a limited amount of time in which to reproduce programmed into them. This theory is supported by the natural slowing down and eventual halting of the processes vital to reproducing and maintaining life which is synonymous with ageing.

Signs of ageing associated with the systemic systems include:

- Loss of short-term memory.
- Gradual loss of special senses e.g. decreasing sight, hearing, taste etc.
- Changes in blood pressure levels resulting in high or low blood pressure.
- A gradual thinning of skin, hair and nails together with a loss of flexibility and lustre.
- A gradual slowing down of the effectiveness in defence mechanisms.

In addition to these natural processes, ageing may be aggravated and indeed speeded up through excessive exposure to certain environmental factors e.g. free radicals. Free radicals are the toxic by-product of energy metabolism and include pollution, radiation and certain foods which are over-processed and/or chemically modified. Free radicals attack individual cells making them less efficient, gradually causing long-term degeneration. Whilst the body has mechanisms to defend against free radical activity, over exposure will result in a deterioration of these defences and an increase in cellular vulnerability.

Reflexology can help the body to maintain more efficient defences through treatment and alert the body to the effects of over-exposure to free radicals through effective aftercare advice.

Awareness

An awareness of the necessity to provide the human body as a whole with the respect it deserves, and a willingness to provide and adapt a level of treatment to meet its needs are the prerequisite of care.

The primary concern of the medical profession is all too often purely associated with life or death – preserving life and avoiding death. Many doctors view the care they offer as being linked solely to these factors without providing access to the care of the many levels of health that come between life and death. The care of a person's well-being at this level then becomes the responsibility of the individual. Complementary treatments are a means to bridge this gap and as such are becoming increasingly popular, with new treatments and adaptations of old treatments constantly emerging.

Reflexology has become widely accepted as one such treatment, with the feet being the most commonly used area for treatment because of their size, location and association with relaxation – most people like having their feet rubbed.

An awareness of the benefits of treating the hands and ears as complementary or alternative sites provides the practitioner with increased treatment possibilities, e.g.

- The reflexes on the fingers are more accessible than those on the toes.
- The reflexes on the hands and ears are more easily accessible for self-treatment.
- Cross-reflexes may be used in the event of contraindicated parts e.g. work the hands instead of the feet.
- Treatment variety maintains client and practitioner interest.

Awareness develops with experience, and experience relies on exploration and discovery. Reflexology demands that one never loses sight of the need to remain aware and to create greater awareness in those we treat.

 Angel advice

A human being will thrive under the spotlight of special care if it has been adapted to meet their needs.

Special care

The adaptation of treatment to meet the needs of each individual client forms the basis for special care.

Special care of the systemic systems of the body will provide the basis for the special care of the rest of the body systems because of their generic links with one another:

- The nervous system communicates the effects of special care to all parts of the body and mind through touch, sight, smell, taste, hearing, intuition etc.
- The blood circulatory system transports the components of such care to every cell i.e. oxygen with improved breathing, water with improved fluid intake, nutrients with improved nutrition.
- The integumentary system provides a mirror image of internal well-being, demonstrating the effects of such care in the external appearance and condition of the hair, skin and nails.
- The immune system responds to special care by providing strengthened defence mechanisms that help to protect every cell, tissue, gland, organ and system of the body.

Special care is an integral part of every treatment and is a multifaceted process which has the potential to provide a domino effect i.e. a cared for person feels more inclined to care for others as well as themselves. In addition, the results of providing special care will often have a knock-on effect on the provider as well as the receiver.

Case study

The human body as a whole relies on the well-being of the systemic systems to maintain its basic functions. If these systems are well, then the other systems have a better chance of being well also. The art of reflexology supports this theory and the skills associated with the reflexology treatment contribute to maintaining well-being. When first studying the art and skill of reflexology, it is important to feel comfortable with all aspects of the treatment including the physical application, the psychological effects on both the client and practitioner and the spiritual use of energy.

This does not happen overnight, nor does it necessarily happen just because you have read a book or attended a course of study. It only happens when you start to live the treatment. It is then that we are able to take on board the complexity and potential of the treatment for both our clients and ourselves.

Initially we may be sceptical about the treatment and its theories, treating every new piece of information with trepidation and in some cases amusement or even an element of fear. This is both normal and healthy and is a view often shared by our clients. It is therefore important to remember these initial feelings as we progress so that we may empathise with other therapists as well as our future clients.

To really start to live the treatment for yourself it is useful to begin by practising the relaxation movements on the feet or hands of family, friends or fellow students. Learn to clear your mind and really feel the effects of your movements. Once you feel your client has reached a level of relaxation whereby they are letting you in you are then able to work to greater depths by treating the systemic systems. Using your thumb or index finger work up and down each longitudinal zone on both hands/feet. Keeping an open mind, start to feel the physical differences as you work over the area. Continue by working in overlapping rows across the transverse zones covering the whole of both feet/hands. You may begin to feel a connection with your client which goes beyond the physical. Trust your instincts and learn to go with the flow. Try to visualise the blood flowing freely through your client's veins and arteries. Imagine the electrical impulses associated with the nervous system being controlled. Observe how the skin of the part you are working on is responding and think about how

▶

Case study (continued)

the effects will spread to the rest of the integumentary system. In your mind's eye start to 'see' the body's natural defences in quiet preparation. Finally, let these positive images spread to all parts of the body as the increased circulation gently feeds every cell, tissue and organ. Finish with some gentle relaxation movements as you bring yourself and your client to the end of the session. You may find that both you and your client have a glazed eye appearance and that the connection between you has intensified. You may also feel drained and emotional. You have been using all of your senses as you learn to truly live your treatment.

Task 1

Think about the consultation considerations for yourself, and after determining your own suitability to the treatment carry out the relaxation techniques described in Chapter 6 on your hands. Using the pressure technique, thumb walk up and down each of the longitudinal and transverse zones. Note the differences as you move along the hand and think about what the effects will be on your general well-being through the treatment of the systemic body systems.

Task 2

After conducting a full consultation, carry out the relaxation and thumb walking techniques on the feet of a friend or colleague. Discuss the treatment in terms of what the feet felt like before, during and after the treatment and what possible effects it will have had on the other body systems as well as the systemic body systems.

When you feel confident on the feet, adapt the techniques for treatment of the hands and ears.

Knowledge review

1   What is the recommended treatment time for a first time client and subsequent treatment?

2   Explain the difference between meiosis and mitosis.

3   What are the three vital resources for life?

4   Give four functions of the human body.

5   Name the four systemic systems of the body.

6   How many cranial and spinal nerves form the peripheral nervous system?

7   Which parts of the autonomic nervous system are responsible for preparing the body for activity and rest?

8   In which direction do arteries and veins transport blood?

9   Name the three layers that make up the skin.

10   Which cells are responsible for defending the body against attack?

Reflexes of the skeletal/muscular systems

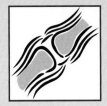

14

Bones and muscles are active living tissue, which are capable of both growth and repair.

Bones are made up of approximately:

- 25 per cent water;
- 45 per cent inorganic materials e.g. calcium and phosphorus; and
- 30 per cent organic substances e.g. osteoblasts (bone-forming cells).

Muscles are made up of approximately:

- 75 per cent water;
- 5 per cent inorganic materials e.g. mineral salts; and
- 20 per cent organic substances e.g. myoblasts (muscle-forming cells).

Bones are soft during childhood allowing for rapid growth, hardening as we age to form solid structures that can withstand a great deal. They contain a combination of **cancellous** and **compact** bone tissue depending on their size, shape and function:

- Cancellous bone tissue is spongy in texture and loose in structure, forming the inner portion of most bones. It contains red bone marrow which is responsible for the formation of new blood cells as well as yellow bone marrow which provides a storage area for fat cells.
- Compact bone tissue is hard in texture and solid in structure providing a covering for cancellous bone tissue.

Tough connective tissue forms an outer covering to most bones in the form of **periosteum** and **cartilage**:

- Periosteum covers the length of bones, producing new bone cells for growth and repair and linking the bones to the circulatory and nervous systems.

- Cartilage covers the ends of bones at a joint, helping to prevent wear and tear as bones move against one another.

Bones form three different types of joints – **fibrous**, **cartilaginous** and **synovial** which are classified according to the amount of movement they allow:

- Fibrous joints are fixed joints allowing no movement between bones; examples include the joints between the bones of the skull in adults.
- Cartilaginous joints are slightly moveable joints which contain pads of cartilage between the bones, allowing only a limited amount of movement; examples include the joints between the bones of the spine.
- Synovial joints are freely moveable joints which are made up of a cavity between the bones containing a fluid allowing ease of movement; examples include the joints of the shoulder, hip, elbow, knee etc.

Bones are linked together at synovial joints by **ligaments**. Also made from tough connective tissue, ligaments allow bones to move freely within a safe range.

Muscles are needed to perform such movements and are attached to bones by **tendons** e.g. the Achilles tendon attaches the calf muscle to the foot at the ankle.

Muscles are made up of fibres which contain thread-like structures called myofibrils extending from one end of the fibre to the other. Each myofibril is made up of a combination of thick and thin threads called myofilaments which work together in much the same way as an extending ladder to form concentric (shortening of the muscle) and eccentric (lengthening of the muscle) contractions.

Also present within the muscle fibres are **mitochondria**. These are responsible for generating the energy needed for the muscle to make a movement, which in turn moves the whole body. Mitochondria are often referred to as powerhouses because they store **glycogen**, **water** and **myoglobin**:

- Glycogen and water are the end products of the carbohydrates, fruit and vegetables we eat and the fluid we drink and are needed to *create* energy.
- Myoglobin holds the oxygen brought to the muscles and is needed to *activate* the energy.

Many functions are expected of the skeletal/muscular systems including shape, support, posture, protection, movement, storage and production.

- The skeleton provides a framework to which the muscles are attached, forming our unique shape.
- Postural muscles maintain the body in an upright position.
- Muscles and bones form a barrier helping to protect the internal organs from external attack.

● The connection between skeletal, visceral and cardiac muscles, bones and the nervous system allow voluntary and involuntary movement associated with vital body functions.

Remember

Skeletal muscles are responsible for voluntary movement, e.g. the hamstrings and quadriceps of the legs when walking. **Visceral** muscles are responsible for the involuntary movements that carry the food through the digestive system etc. and **cardiac** muscles are associated with the movement of the heart.

● Bones take organic matter from the blood i.e. minerals and fat to be stored.
● Red bone marrow produces new blood cells and muscle movement produces heat.

We rely on the efficient working of the skeletal/muscular systems throughout life, often taking their functions for granted. As a result, the systems become stressed and fail to perform effectively. Underuse of the systems is equally distressing to their well-being as over activity with wasted muscles and bones resulting from the former and aching, fatigued muscles and joints from the latter. If such symptoms are ignored, further degeneration develops as other body systems become involved. Reflexology provides an holistic approach to the well-being of the muscular/skeletal systems and, as a result, of the body as a whole.

Remember

The body systems do not work in isolation – they rely on each other for their continued well-being.

System sorter

SKELETAL/MUSCULAR SYSTEMS

Nervous system
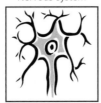

Skeletal muscles are attached to bones at joints by tendons. Motor nerves enter the muscle at a motor point branching out to supply each muscle fibre with a motor end plate. Stimulation of the motor point by the brain in response to a stimulus alerts the muscle to contract, pulling the bones like levers in order to perform a specific movement.

Circulatory system

The blood transports oxygen, glycogen and water to the muscles for the production of energy and transports the waste products associated with energy production away to be excreted out of the body. Red bone marrow is found in cancellous bone tissue and is responsible for the formation of new blood cells.

Integumentary system
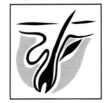

Vitamin D is produced in the skin in response to sunlight and helps the bones absorb calcium, which is needed to keep them strong and healthy. A lack of vitamin D in children results in the malformation of bone tissue associated with rickets. The skin also contributes to temperature control by releasing sweat onto its surface when muscles are producing excessive heat due to overexertion.

Immune system
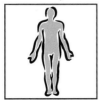

Non-specific defence mechanisms include the process of phagocytosis. Special cells called phagocytes engulf foreign particles, micro-organisms e.g. bacteria, viruses, fungi etc. and old cells helping to protect the body against disease. Phagocytosis occurs in the bones and muscles to remove damaged tissue associated with injury, thus helping to prevent further problems.

Cells

Osteoblasts are bone-forming cells and myoblasts are muscle-forming cells. The develoment of bones is continuous throughout life with bones reaching a certain thickness, length and shape when a person has reached the age of 25. Muscles contain a combination of slow- and fast-twitch fibres allowing varied movement. Slow-twitch fibres produce slow contractions for a long time; fast-twitch fibres produce rapid contraction for only a short time.

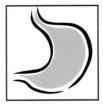

The bones and muscles of the thorax protect the respiratory organs and contribute to the depth of breathing. In turn the respiratory system provides the bones and muscles with oxygen for growth, repair and production of energy in order to perform a movement.

Respiratory system
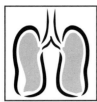

Any excess calcium and phosphorus in the body that is not stored in the bones, together with waste products from energy production in the muscles, is excreted from the body in urine.

Genito-urinary system

Hormones are responsible for controlling the growth rate in bones and changes in muscles during puberty. They are also responsible for the decline in bone and muscle density associated with ageing e.g. menopause in women and andropause in men.

Endocrine system
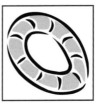

The main lymph nodes of the body are located at specific points within the skeletal/muscular systems. Axillary nodes are found within the shoulder girdle, the supratrochlear nodes are found at the elbow, the inguinal within the pelvic girdle and the popliteal nodes behind the knee. These nodes are responsible for filtering fluid lymph, thus removing toxins from the cells.

Lymphatic system
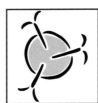

Nutrients from the food we eat are broken down in the digestive system. Carbohydrates are broken down into glycogen and transported to the muscles via the blood where they are needed for energy production. Calcium and phosphorus are transported to the skeleton where they are needed for strong, healthy bones.

Digestive system

Consultation considerations

In order to ascertain the level of stress the skeletal/muscular systems are under, it is useful to consider the following during the consultation process.

Oral

When questioning the client, it is advisable to include questions that provide an insight into the activity affecting the bones and muscles e.g.

- Profession – a person's job will help to determine the amount of strain put on the systems and whether or not their work entails repetitive strenuous activity that may be responsible for any symptoms they are experiencing,

- History of injury – a past fracture, tear or sprain may result in a general weakness in the corresponding bones, joints and muscles.

- Exercise – the amount and type of exercise will determine the amount of under- or overuse of the systems.

Visual

When observing the client it is necessary to take note of the following factors:

- Shape and size – the shape and size of the whole skeletal/muscular structure will provide an insight into the person type, as will the shape of the part e.g. foot, hand or ear. In addition, shape and size of individual muscles denotes tone and flexibility.

- Gait – the way in which the client walks provides an insight into the well-being of the skeletal/muscular systems and as a result, the well-being of the body as a whole due to the links between the systems.

- Posture – overall well-being and specific areas of stress can be seen in the way in which a person holds themselves upright. Poor posture results in imbalance between opposing muscle groups and postural faults which in turn lead to aching and fatigued muscles and strained joints.

In addition, the skeletal/muscular systems are responsible for the movements associated with body language. Physical and emotional pain is often reflected in closed body language and pained facial expressions.

Aural

It is not only important to hear the words a client is saying but also to listen to the meaning behind the words, e.g. pain is often expressed as anger and frustration. In addition other factors may be heard including:

- Creaking joints – denoting a loss of free movement in muscles and joints.
- Cracking joints – denoting changes in pressure within a joint.

Olfactory

The use of all of our senses can provide the key to an effective consultation and the sense of smell can alert us to additional problems associated with a person's physical and emotional well-being, e.g. feelings of worthlessness may be accompanied by a lack of personal hygiene etc.

Perceptive

A general sense of the client may be picked up intuitively by the practitioner during the consultation. The way in which people hold themselves by using their skeletal/muscular systems helps to determine their levels of self-worth. The willingness to open up may also be perceived through a person's muscular/skeletal system e.g. a closed-in framework denotes a closed-in attitude etc.

Tactile

The art of touch can provide a useful tool when analysing the skeletal/muscular systems by actually touching the muscles in question and/or the corresponding parts of the feet, hands or ears to determine the levels of stress felt in each area.

- Good tone can be felt in firm muscles and freely moveable joints.
- Poor tone can be felt in flaccid muscles and creaking joints.
- Fatigue can be felt in tight muscles and tight joints.

Angel advice

Care should be taken when treating the very young and the elderly. Bone tissue is still developing in the very young and bones may become brittle in the elderly. Movements should be applied with gentle pressure to avoid damage.

Contraindication considerations

It is not advisable to work directly over any reflexes associated with the skeletal/muscular system that are excessively painful or swollen. Whilst it is okay to work over stressed areas to relieve tension, working over areas of distress may aggravate the condition. If this is the case, consider working the hands instead of the feet, the ears instead of the hands etc.

It is also possible to consider working the cross-referral areas associated with the individual reflex e.g. if the reflex for the hip is too painful to work try the reflex for the shoulder etc.

Reflexes

Working over the whole of the feet, hands and/or ears affects the *general* overall well-being of these systems as muscles and bones form many parts of the body. Isolating and treating *specific* reflex points associated with these systems highlights those areas that are affected by excessive stress and strain.

The axial skeleton

Comprises:

- The skull – the cranium and the face.
- The spine – the neck and back.
- The thorax – the chest.

The skull

Comprises the bones of the cranium and of the face, the joints of which are fibrous (allowing no movement) except for the lower jaw which is a synovial joint (allowing free movement associated with talking and eating). Covering the surface of the skull are muscles, skin and hair, which are all linked by the circulatory systems. The skull acts as protection for the underlying organ of the central nervous system – the brain. The brain contains the pituitary and pineal endocrine glands as well as the hypothalamus linking the endocrine and nervous systems together. Twelve pairs of cranial nerves radiate out from the brain to all areas of the face and neck. Together these nerves supply the sense organs (skin, eyes, ears, nose and tongue) and muscles with the ability to sense a stimulus and respond by sending messages in the form of impulses to and from the brain. Working over this whole area will have an affect on all of these structures which will in turn affect the rest of the body.

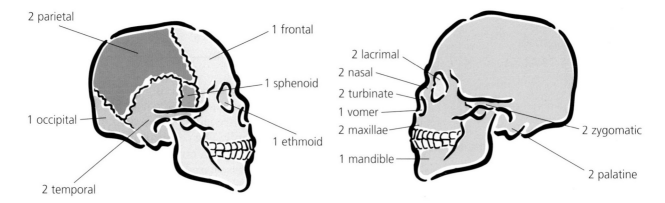

Bones of the cranium

2 parietal
1 frontal
1 sphenoid
1 occipital
1 ethmoid
2 temporal

Bones of the face

2 lacrimal
2 nasal
2 turbinate
1 vomer
2 maxillae
1 mandible
2 zygomatic
2 palatine

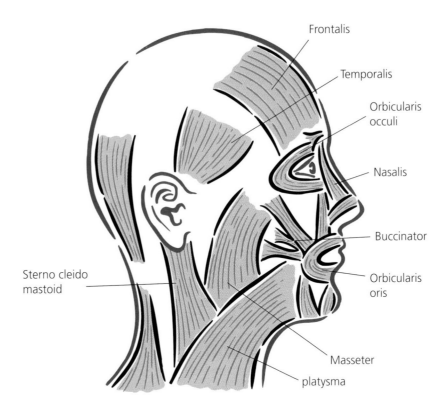

Muscles of the cranium and face

The spine

Consists of five sections of vertebrae held together by either synovial, cartilaginous or fibrous joints. In addition, muscles, skin and hair, blood and lymph service the area. The whole of the spine protects the underlying spinal cord, from which 31 pairs of spinal nerves radiate to form plexuses and branch out to provide nerves to all parts of the body.

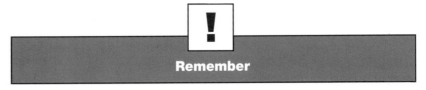

Remember

A **plexus** is simply a network of nerves.

Seven cervical vertebrae form the neck and upper section of the back. The first two vertebrae are joined at synovial joints allowing movement of the head. The rest are joined at cartilaginous joints allowing restricted movement only. The cervical plexus contains the first four cervical nerves which branch out to supply the neck and shoulder. The phrenic nerve is associated with this plexus and stimulates the contraction of the diaphragm during breathing.

Twelve thoracic vertebrae form the upper and mid-back to which theribs are attached. The joints in this section of the back are all

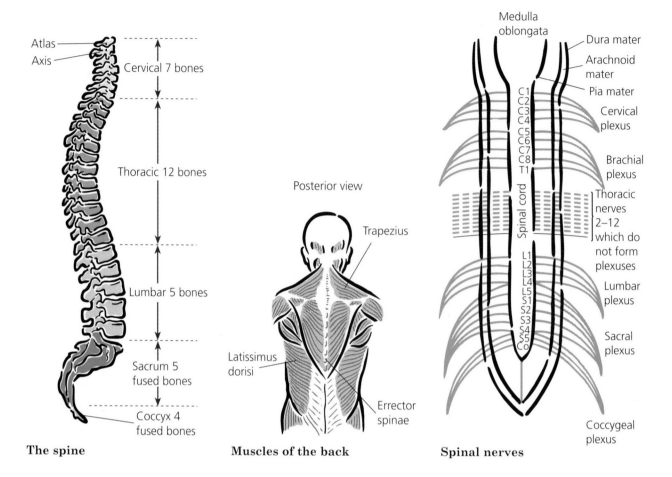

The spine

Muscles of the back

Spinal nerves

cartilaginous. The brachial plexus contains the remaining four cervical nerves and part of the first thoracic nerve to supply the arms.

The rest of the thoracic nerves do not form a plexus but instead provide an individual nerve supply to the chest and abdomen.

Five lumbar vertebrae form the lower back. The joints in this section are also cartilaginous. The lumbar plexus contains the first three lumbar nerves and part of the fourth which supply the lower abdomen, groin and part of the legs.

Five sacral vertebrae form the base of the back. The bones are fused together forming fibrous joints with no movement. The sacral plexus contains part of the fourth lumbar nerve, the fifth and the

Remember

The sciatic nerve is the longest nerve of the body, extending from the sacral plexus to the feet and is one that is often affected by physical stress, causing the pain and discomfort associated with sciatica.

first four sacral nerves to supply the pelvis, the buttocks and part of the legs. The sciatic nerve is one of the nerves that branches out from this plexus.

Four coccyx bones form the tail. These bones are also fused together forming fibrous joints.

The coccygeal plexus contains part of the fourth and fifth sacral nerves and the coccygeal nerves to supply the external structures of the digestive and reproductive organs.

The thorax

Made up of the thoracic vertebrae of the back to which 12 pairs of ribs are attached. The joints are synovial, offering a gliding movement, which enables the chest to expand during breathing. The first seven ribs attach at the front of the body to the sternum (breastbone), the next three to the ribs above them and the final two pairs of ribs are classed as floating as they do not attach to anything at the front of the body. The bones of the thorax are covered with muscles including the muscles of the chest, i.e. pectorals, and those associated with breathing, i.e. intercostals.

Remember

The diaphragm is a dome-shaped sheet of muscle forming the internal divide between the organs of the chest, i.e. heart and lungs and the abdominal organs. When contracted the diaphragm pushes the abdominal organs downwards to allow the lungs to increase in size as they inflate during inspiration.

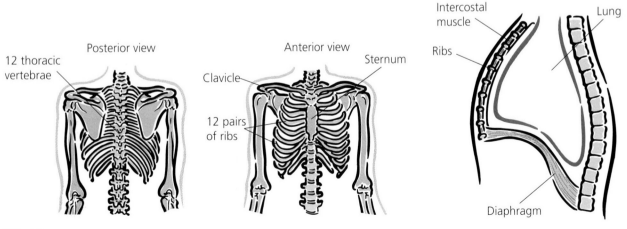

The thorax

The bones and muscles of the thorax provide the heart and lungs with protection, which is further enhanced by the overlying skin. The circulatory systems service the area with blood and lymph and the nervous system controls the rate of breathing and associated muscular action.

The appendicular skeleton

Comprises:

- The shoulder girdle, arms and hands.
- The pelvic girdle, legs and feet.

The shoulder girdle offers additional protection to the heart and lungs, whilst the pelvic girdle protects the lower abdominal organs. These areas form the majority of the synovial (freely) moveable joints of the body i.e. the shoulder, elbow, wrist, hip, knee and ankle and are worked as a whole.

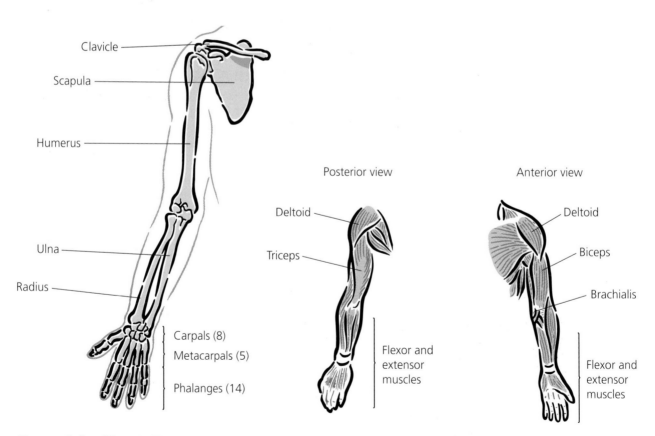

Bones of shoulder girdle and arms   **Muscles of shoulder girdle and arms**

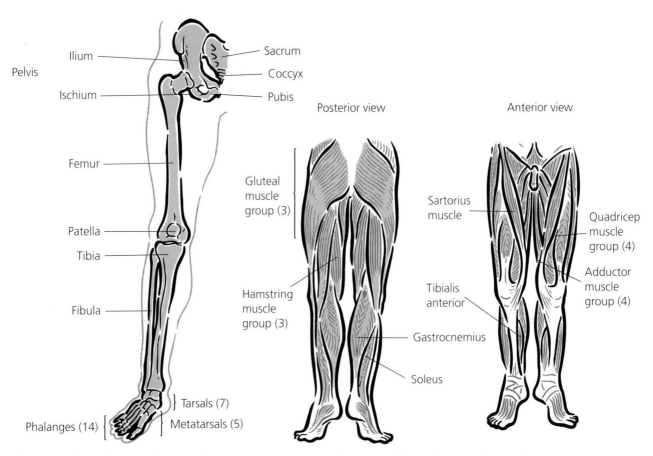

Bones of the pelvic girdle and legs

Muscles of the pelvic girdle and legs

The position of the reflexes

The whole of the big toe, thumb and ear lobe relates to the head.

- Back of the head – plantar aspect of the big toe and palmar surface of the thumb and the earlobe.
- Face including eyes, nose and mouth – dorsal aspect of the big toe and thumb and the earlobe.
- Neck – base of big toe and thumb and the base of the antihelix.
- Brain/ears/cranial nerves – top and sides of big toe and thumb and along the tragus and antitragus of the ear.
- Spine – along the medial edge of the feet/hands from the base of the big toe/thumb nail down to the pelvic line and the medial edge of the antihelix from the antitragus to the medial edge of the helix of the ears.
- Sternum – directly below the big toe/thumb on the dorsal aspect of the feet and hands.
- Ribs – from zones 1–5 along the dorsal aspect of the feet and hands. The thorax is located in the antihelix region of the ear in line with the thoracic vertebrae.
- Joints – along the lateral edge of the feet and hands and the antihelix of the ears.

Tip

There is much controversy surrounding the exact position of the joint reflexes on the feet and hands and whilst the position of the shoulder and hip reflexes is logical, those of the elbow, knee, wrist and ankle are not quite so clear.

- Some practitioners take the view that the position of the shoulder and hip reflexes incorporates the reflexes for the elbow and wrist and knee and ankle respectively.

- Others believe that the joints follow a logical order as if the hand were hanging to the side of the body tracking the shoulder, elbow, hip and wrist down. This leaves no room for the knee and ankle which are sometimes believed to be worked as cross-reflexes when working the elbow or wrist.

Remember

A cross-reflex refers to the areas of the body that are anatomically related, e.g. elbow and knee, wrist and ankle, and may also be classified as referral reflexes or zones.

- Another view states that the feet and hands represent the body in a foetal position. As such the wrist and shoulder reflexes and the elbow, hip and ankle reflexes would be located together with the knee in between the two areas.

- A further view is that the arms and legs cannot be specifically located within the feet and hands as these areas are only able to represent those parts of the body we cannot live without i.e. the head and trunk.

Angel advice

Experience will heighten your perception and you will eventually be able to make up your own mind as to the location of these specific reflexes.

Skeletal/muscular systems – order of work

Tip

It is worth noting that clients often experience a tingling sensation in a limb when the spinal reflexes are being worked and this can be logically linked with the corresponding nerve.

Tip

Working the spine and head also works the seven chakras.

Remember

The sciatic nerve is the longest nerve of the body, extending from the sacral plexus to the feet.

Tip

Chronic sciatica can be helped by lifting and supporting the leg with one hand and with the other hand giving a slow sliding and pinching movement to the midline of the calf from ankle up – as far as is comfortable.

Suggested order of work – feet

Using the thumb or index finger to work/stimulate the area and/or sliding movements to soothe the area:

- *Cranium* – work up the plantar aspect (underside) of the big toe from the base to the tip in small overlapping rows. Work over until the whole of the area has been covered.
- *Face* – proceed down the dorsal (top) aspect of the big toe from the base of the nail to the base of the toe in small overlapping rows. Work over until the whole area has been covered.
- *Neck* – work along the base of the big toe from the medial edge of both the dorsal and plantar aspects of the foot. Repeat twice more.
- *Top and sides* – work up the side of the big toe, over the top and down the other side.
- *Spine* – work down the medial (inner) edge of the foot starting from just below the nail area on the big toe. Follow the curve of the foot, feeling for the bones. Work down to the pelvic line.
- Repeat the movement upwards from pelvic line to big toe.
- Repeat the complete movement twice more counting the individual vertebrae as you work downwards – 7 cervical, 12 thoracic, 5 lumbar, sacrum and coccyx.

By working over the spinal reflexes all of the 31 pairs of nerves will be treated, however, in addition to this, the sciatic nerve has its own reflex areas.

- *Sciatic nerve* – work across the heel of the foot just under the pelvic line. Start at zone 1 through to zone 5 and slide back. Repeat using other hand from zone 5 to zone 1.
- *Thorax* – using the index finger, work along the dorsal (top) aspect of the foot from the gap in between the base of each toe to the middle of the foot. Slide back up and repeat twice more.

Tip

The sternum is located along the medial aspect of the area directly below the big toe.

- *Joints* – work down the lateral (outer) edge of the feet starting from just below the nail area on the little toe. Follow the curve of the foot feeling for the bones. Work down to the base of the feet. Repeat twice more.
- The shoulder, elbow, wrist, hip, knee and ankle joints will all be worked. Corresponding muscles, tendons and ligaments will also be aided as will blood and lymph.

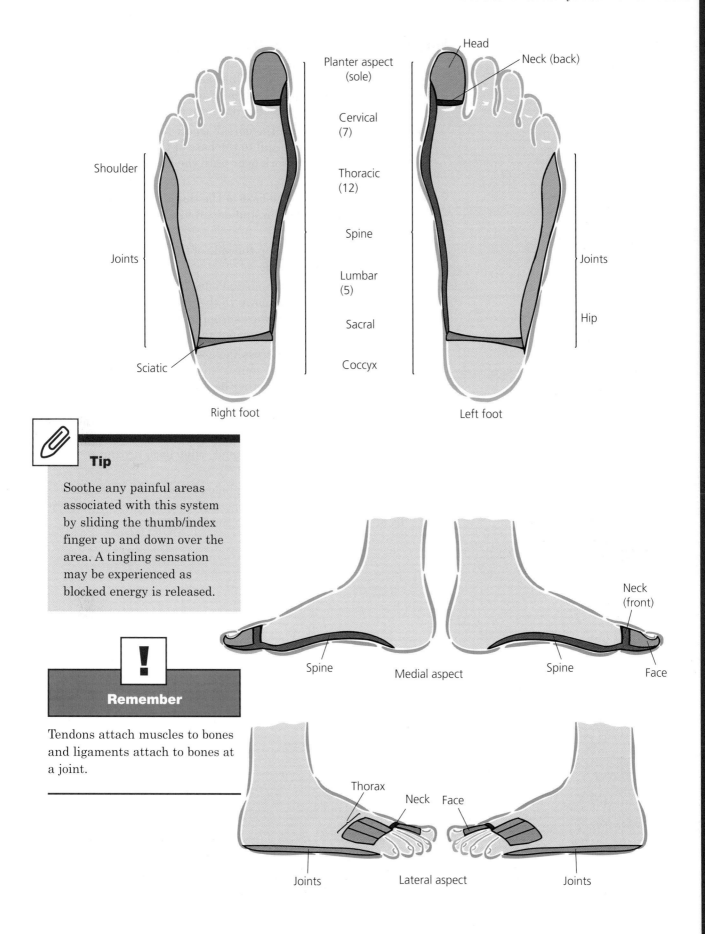

Right foot

Left foot

Planter aspect (sole)

Cervical (7)

Thoracic (12)

Spine

Lumbar (5)

Sacral

Coccyx

Shoulder

Joints

Sciatic

Head

Neck (back)

Joints

Hip

Tip

Soothe any painful areas associated with this system by sliding the thumb/index finger up and down over the area. A tingling sensation may be experienced as blocked energy is released.

!

Remember

Tendons attach muscles to bones and ligaments attach to bones at a joint.

Spine

Medial aspect

Spine

Neck (front)

Face

Thorax

Neck   Face

Joints

Lateral aspect

Joints

Suggested order of work – hands

- *Cranium* – work up the palmar aspect of the thumb from the base to the tip in small overlapping rows. Work over until the whole of the area has been covered.
- *Face* – proceed down the dorsal aspect (top) of the thumb from the base of the nail to the base of the thumb in small overlapping rows. Work over until the whole of the area has been covered.
- *Neck* – work along the base of the thumb from the medial edge of both the palmar and dorsal aspects of the hand. Repeat twice more.
- *Top and sides* – work up the side of the thumb, over the top and down the other side.
- *Spine* – work down the medial edge of the hand from the base of the thumbnail down to the pelvic line. Repeat the movement working upwards from pelvic line to thumb. Repeat the complete movement twice more.
- *Sciatic nerve* – work across the heel of the hand just under the pelvic line. Start at zone 1 through to zone 5 and slide back. Repeat using the other hand, working from zone 5 to zone 1.
- *Thorax* – using the index finger, work along the dorsal aspect of the hand from the gap in between the base of each finger to the middle of the hand. Slide back up and repeat twice more.
- *Joints* – using the thumb or index finger work down the lateral edge of the hand. Repeat the movement, working up from the base of the hand to the little finger.

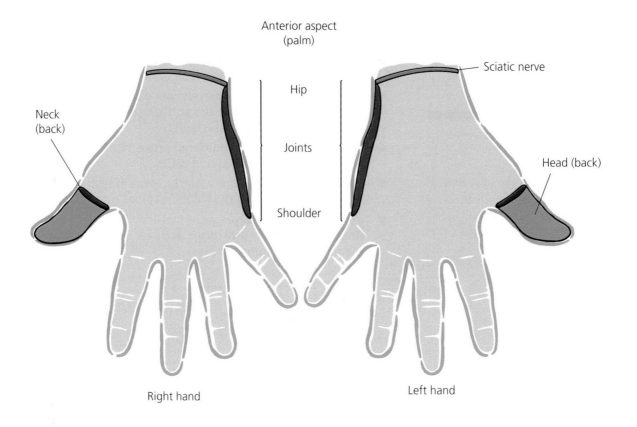

Anterior aspect
(palm)

Sciatic nerve

Hip

Joints

Shoulder

Neck
(back)

Head (back)

Right hand

Left hand

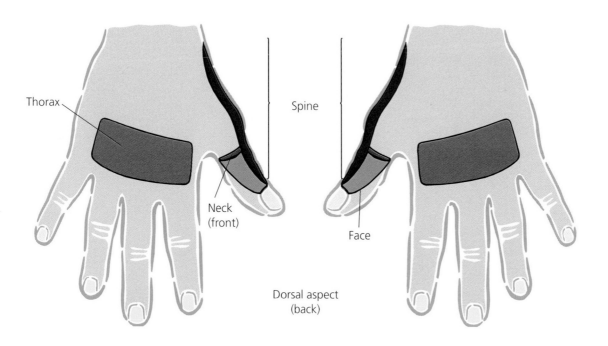

Thorax

Spine

Neck
(front)

Face

Dorsal aspect
(back)

Suggested order of work – ears

- *Head and face* – small pressure movements using thumb and index finger over the whole of the ear lobe.
- *Spine* – small pressure movements using the index finger along the medial edge of the antihelix from the antitragus to the medial aspect of the helix.
- *Sciatic nerve* – Apply additional pressure on the antihelix in line with the sacral spinal reflex.
- *Thorax* – apply pressure with the index finger along the antihelix in line with the thoracic spinal reflex.
- *Joints* – apply small pressure movements with the index finger to the upper and lower portions of the antihelix including the triangular fossa.

Tip

The joints are well represented on the ears and access to the knee, elbow, ankle and wrist may be easier than those on the hands or feet.

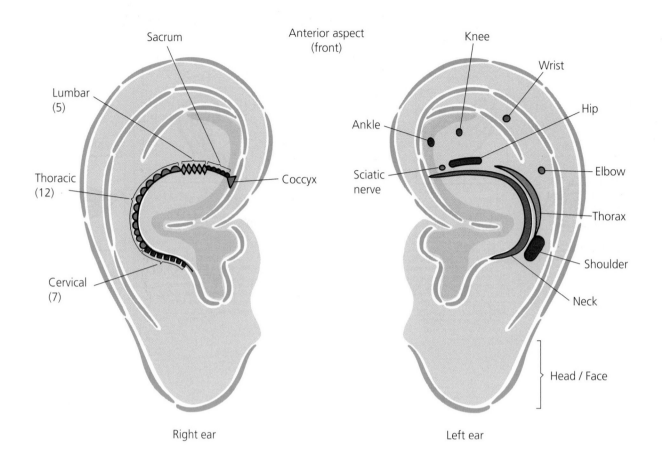

Sacrum

Anterior aspect
(front)

Knee

Lumbar
(5)

Wrist

Ankle

Hip

Thoracic
(12)

Coccyx

Sciatic
nerve

Elbow

Thorax

Cervical
(7)

Shoulder

Neck

Head / Face

Right ear

Left ear

Treatment tracker

SKELETAL/MUSCULAR SYSTEMS

Hands

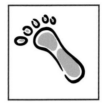

Feet

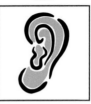

Ears

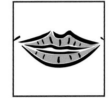

Visualisation

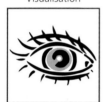

Affirmation

The use of visualisation can help to reduce the build-up of tension in the skeletal/muscular systems as a result of unsafe stress. This will have a knock-on effect on the rest of the body, mind and spirit. Try to visualise the rays of the sun bathing the whole of the body in warmth. Imagine the feeling as the tight muscles soften and loosen and any troubled thoughts appear to melt away in the heat. Now try to visualise a cool breeze maintaining just the perfect temperature as you continue to bathe in the afterglow.

The skull is located on the thumb, the spine along the medial edge, the thorax on the dorsal aspect and the major synovial joints along the lateral edge of the hand. The reflexes for the associated joints and muscles are located according to the position of the bones to which they connect. The hands provide an ideal site for self-treatment of the skeletal/muscular systems, helping to ease tense muscles and tight joints.

The skull is located on the big toe, the spine on the medial edge, the thorax on the dorsal aspect and the major synovial joints along the lateral edge of the feet. The reflexes for the associated joints and muscles are located according to the position of the bones to which they connect. Because of their size the feet provide greater access to these reflexes, thus helping to promote maximum benefit to these systems.

The skull is located on the lobe of the ear, the spine along the base of the antihelix and the thorax and major synovial joints are located within the antihelix. The reflexes for the associated muscles and joints are located according to the position of the bones to which they connect. The ears provide an ideal, easily identifiable site for the treatment of the reflexes of the limbs.

An affirmation for the skeletal/muscular system should reflect the systems' functions. The ability to function well will be reflected in the well-being of the systems and that of the whole body. 'My life is whole, I am supported, I am flexible and I am able to move freely.' This in turn helps a person to relate such a thought to all aspects of their lives, instilling positive thinking where sometimes the negativity associated with stress takes over.

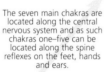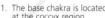

All colours may be linked with the skeletal/muscular systems depending on the position of the bones and muscles in the body and the associated organs they protect.
An interesting use of colour is to ask a client to choose a colour from an array of different coloured towels, crystals and gemstones or alternatively to open their mind and see which colour enters it. Their choice of colour will reflect their physical and emotional needs; by working with that colour the potential effectiveness of the treatment is increased. The use of crystals and gemstones provides an exciting and interesting way of developing the use of colour for aftercare.

The seven main chakras are located along the central nervous system and as such chakras one–five can be located along the spine reflexes on the feet, hands and ears.

1. The base chakra is located at the coccyx region.
2. The sacral chakra is located at the sacral region.
3. The solar plexus chakra is located at the lumbar region.
4. The heart chakra is located at the thoracic region.
5. The throat chakra is located at the base of the cervical region.

The sixth and seventh, brow and crown chakras can be found in the reflexes for the head.
Treatment over these areas will help to balance the energy flow within the whole of the body as well as in each individual chakra.

The skeletal/muscular systems can be found in all of the five longitudinal zones of the feet and hands.

● The spine is located in zone 1.
● The shoulder and pelvic girdles and the thorax are all located in zones 1–5.
● The major synovial joints are located in zone 5.

The skeletal/muscular systems can also be found in each of the transverse zones in the feet, hands and ears.

The 12 main meridians all form channels of energy which have an effect on the well-being of the skeletal/muscular systems. The natural ebb and flow of energy within the meridians contributes to the stimulation and sedation of the skeletal/muscular systems and a balance must be maintained if these systems are to function well. All forms of complementary treatment can help to control this free flow of energy, helping to unblock areas of congestion, thus maintaining the functions of the body as a whole.

The notes D and A are linked with the skeletal/muscular systems:

● The note D affects the skeletal system, and music that is flowing is most suitable to balance the system, encouraging ease of movement.
● The note A affects the muscular system and any form of classical music is suitable to balance the system and encourage freedom of movement.

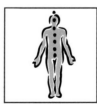

Colour

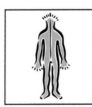

Chakras

Zones

Meridians

Sound

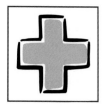

Common conditions

When treating problems associated with the skeletal/muscular system it is always advisable to complete a full treatment to include all reflexes, paying particular attention to those *directly* affecting the problem as well as those indirectly involved.

As stress is often the cause and/or a contributory factor in most problems affecting these systems, attention should be paid to the pituitary and adrenal glands for their role in the body's response to stress. The solar plexus reflex (see the respiratory system, Chapter 15) will need extra attention due to its de-stressing function. Particular attention should also be paid to the elimination reflexes of the body e.g. lymphatic nodes and ducts (see the lymphatic system, Chapter 19), kidneys, ureters and bladder (see the genito-urinary system, Chapter 17) for their role in ridding the body of the waste products associated with stress. The list below gives common conditions of the skeletal/muscular systems together with direct and indirect reflexes.

An A–Z of common conditions affecting the skeletal/muscular systems

 Activity

Working through each condition, try to analyse the reasons for paying particular attention to the indirect reflexes. Refer to the reflexes for the appropriate body systems within the other parts of this chapter for more information. This activity will help you to become more aware of the bigger picture associated with good health rather than the smaller picture that is often associated with individual symptoms.

- ANKYLOSING SPONDYLITIS – a disease of the joints usually affecting the spine, resulting in back pain and stiffness. *Direct reflex* = affected area e.g. the spine. *Indirect reflexes* = lungs, chest, parathyroid glands, shoulders, hips, knee.
- ARTHRITIS – inflammation of the joints. Arthritis may be acute or chronic. *Direct reflex* = affected area. *Indirect reflexes* = spine, parathyroid glands.
- ATROPHY – wasting of muscle tissue. *Direct reflex* = affected area e.g. the arm, leg etc. *Indirect reflex* = associated joints.
- BURSITIS – the bursa becomes inflamed and affects the movement within the joint. When this disorder affects the knee it is known as housemaid's knee. *Direct reflex* = affected area e.g. the knee *Indirect reflexes* = associated joints.
- CARTILAGE, torn – a knee injury resulting from sudden twisting movements tearing the cartilage that lies between the joints. *Direct reflex* = affected area e.g. the knee. *Indirect reflexes* = associated joints.
- COCCYNYNIA – pain in the base of the spine usually occurring after injury to the coccyx bone. *Direct reflex* = coccyx region of the spine. *Indirect reflexes* = other areas of the spine, legs.
- CRAMP – a sudden involuntary contraction of a muscle causing acute pain. *Direct reflex* = affected area. *Indirect reflexes* = spine, parathyroid glands.

- FATIGUE – build up of lactic acid in the muscle causing loss of use. *Direct reflex* = affected area. *Indirect reflex* = small intestines, lungs.
- FIBROSITIS – inflammation of the muscle fibres. *Direct reflex* = affected area. *Indirect reflexes* = associated joints.
- FRACTURE – a break or a crack in a bone due to injury, repeated stress to a bone or weakened bone caused by disease. *Direct reflex* = affected area. *Indirect reflexes* = associated joints, parathyroid glands, thyroid glands, spleen.
- FROZEN SHOULDER – a severe aching pain in the shoulder affecting the middle-aged and elderly, which restricts shoulder movements. *Direct reflex* = shoulder. *Indirect reflexes* = spine, arm, neck.
- GANGLION – a harmless swelling at a tendon near a joint. Usually found on the hands or feet. *Direct reflex* = affected area. *Indirect reflexes* = associated joints.
- GOUT – pain in the joints, particularly the big toe, are a symptom of this condition which is an upset of the chemical processes of the body. Knees, ankles, wrists and elbows may also be affected. *Direct reflex* = affected area. *Indirect reflexes* = associated joints.
- KYPHOSIS – concave curve of the spine in the thoracic region creating a humpback and rounded shoulders. *Direct reflex* = thoracic spine. *Indirect reflexes* = the rest of the spine, shoulder, chest, lungs.
- LORDOSIS – convex curve of the spine in the lumbar region creating a hollow back. *Direct reflex* = lumbar spine. *Indirect reflexes* = the rest of the spine, hip joint, legs.
- MUSCULAR DYSTROPHIES – inherited diseases resulting in the collapse of muscle leading to loss of function. *Direct reflex* = affected area. *Indirect reflexes* = associated joints, spine, head.
- MYALGIA – muscle pain. *Direct reflex* = affected area. *Indirect reflexes* = associated joints, thyroid gland, pituitary gland.
- MYASTHENIA GRAVIS – chronic disease in which muscles are weak and tire easily. *Direct reflex* = affected area. *Indirect reflexes* = associated joints, eyes, jaws, throat, lungs, thymus gland.
- MYOKYMIA – persistent quivering of muscles. *Direct reflex* = affected area. *Indirect reflexes* = parathyroid glands, thyroid gland, pituitary gland.
- MYOMA – tumour composed of muscular and fibrous tissue. Commonly found in or on the uterus. *Direct reflex* = affected area. *Indirect reflexes* = fallopian tubes, ovaries.
- MYOSITIS – inflammation of skeletal muscle. *Direct reflex* = affected area. *Indirect reflexes* = associated joints.
- MYOTONIA – prolonged muscular spasms. *Direct reflex* = affected area. *Indirect reflexes* = associated joints, parathyroid glands, thyroid gland, pituitary gland.

- OSTEOARTHRITIS – a degenerative disease of the joints. The cartilage within the joints wears away resulting in pain. Extreme cases result in a joint replacement e.g. the hip, knee etc. *Direct reflex* = affected area e.g. the hip. *Indirect reflexes* = associated joints e.g. the knees etc. spine, parathyroid glands, thyroid gland, pituitary gland.
- OSTEOCHONDRITIS – softening of bone, causing the bone to change shape resulting in deformed bones. Affects children. *Direct reflex* = affected area. *Indirect reflexes* = associated joints, spine, parathyroid glands, thyroid gland, pituitary gland.
- OSTEOGENESIS – defect of the bone cells causing brittle bones. A blue tinge to the eyes often accompanies this condition. *Direct reflex* = affected area. *Indirect reflexes* = associated joints, spine, parathyroid glands, thyroid gland, pituitary gland, eyes,
- OSTEOMALACIA, rickets – softening of bone due to lack of Vitamin D. *Direct reflex* = affected area e.g. the legs. *Indirect reflexes* = associated joints, spine, parathyroid glands, thyroid gland, pituitary gland.
- OSTEOMYELITIS – Inflammation of the bone caused by a bacterial infection, often as a result of a localised injury. *Direct reflex* = affected area. *Indirect reflexes* = associated joints.
- OSTEOPOROSIS – weakening of the bones, which may be caused by changing levels of the hormones oestrogen and progesterone. *Direct reflex* = affected area. *Indirect reflexes* = ovaries, pituitary gland.
- PAGET'S DISEASE OF THE BONES – thickening of the bones causing pain and broadening of bone. *Direct reflex* = affected area. *Indirect reflexes* = spine, head, parathyroid glands, thyroid gland, pituitary gland.
- PARALYSIS – loss of ability to move a part of the body. *Direct reflex* = affected area. *Indirect reflexes* = spine, neck, head.
- PARESIS – partial or slight paralysis of muscles. *Direct reflex* = affected area. *Indirect reflexes* = spine, neck, head.
- RHEUMATOID ARTHRITIS – a destructive swelling of the joints affecting the fingers and feet first but spreading to the wrists, knees, shoulders, ankles and elbows. *Direct reflex* = affected area e.g. the wrists. *Indirect reflexes* = spine.
- RUPTURE – tearing of the muscle fascia or tendon. *Direct reflex* = affected area. *Indirect reflexes* = associated joints.
- SCIATICA – abnormal pressure on any part of the length of the sciatic nerve, which extends down the legs from the lower back, resulting in pain. *Direct reflex* = sciatic nerve. *Indirect reflexes* = spine, hip, knee and ankle.
- SCOLIOSIS – a lateral (away from the midline) curve in the spine. *Direct reflex* = affected area of the spine. *Indirect reflexes* = other areas of the spine, associated joints.

- SHIN SPLINTS – soreness in the front of the lower leg caused by excess walking up and down steps or a hill. *Direct reflex* = lower leg. *Indirect reflexes* = associated joints e.g. ankles and knees.
- SPASM – a sudden involuntary muscle contraction. *Direct reflex* = affected area. *Indirect reflexes* = associated joints.
- SPRAIN – a sudden stretching or tearing of a ligament resulting in pain and swelling. *Direct reflex* = affected area. *Indirect reflexes* = associated joints.
- SLIPPED DISC – a bulging of one of the fibrocartilage discs that separate the vertebrae, causing pain and muscle weakness. *Direct reflex* = affected area of the spine. *Indirect reflexes* = other areas of the spine, associated joints e.g. shoulder, hip.
- STRAIN – overuse of muscles. *Direct reflex* = affected area. *Indirect reflexes* = associated joints.
- STRESS – stiff joints, muscular tension and repetitive strain injury are symptoms of the effect of excessive stress on the skeletal/muscular systems. *Direct reflex* = affected area. *Indirect reflexes* = adrenal glands, pituitary glands, solar plexus, liver, kidneys, spine, head.
- SYNOVITIS – inflammation of a joint after injury. *Direct reflex* = affected area. *Indirect reflexes* = associated joints.
- TENDINITIS – inflammation of tendon and muscle attachments. *Direct reflex* = affected area. *Indirect reflexes* = associated joints.
- TENOSYNOVITIS – inflammation of a tendon sheath where it passes over a joint. *Direct reflex* = affected area. *Indirect reflexes* = associated joints.
- TORTICOLLIS – involuntary contraction of the muscles of the neck. Also known as WRYNECK. *Direct reflex* = the neck. *Indirect reflexes* = other areas of the spine, head, shoulder, arm.
- WHIPLASH – backward jerking of the neck resulting in damage to the spine. *Direct reflex* = the neck. *Indirect reflexes* = other areas of the spine, head, shoulder, arm, chest.

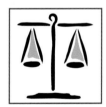

Holistic harmony

The skeletal/muscular systems are a complex network of organs that contribute to the external and internal well-being of the body as a whole. The skeleton provides us with a basic shape to which muscles are added, forming a framework that identifies us as being part of the human race, but at the same time distinguishes us from other people because of our own individual physical characteristics. The skeletal/muscular systems maintain vital links with all of the other systems to ensure that their functions can take place efficiently and effectively. Without this link, the quest for homeostasis would be impossible. It is useful to explore the external factors that affect the maintenance of the body's continuous quest for balance and harmony in relation to the skeletal/muscular systems.

Air

Bones and muscles need a good supply of oxygen to keep them in good working order. Oxygen is needed to feed bones and muscles and activate the energy required to perform the chemical reactions in order for the skeletal/muscular systems to function. The air we breathe is a mixture of gases including approximately 78 per cent nitrogen, 21 per cent oxygen and 1 per cent of other gases e.g. carbon dioxide. This air also contains varying amounts of moisture, dust and pollutants. Airborne pollutants aggravate these functions and contribute to the conditions that affect the skeletal/muscular systems e.g. rheumatoid arthritis and osteoarthritis.

The bones and skeletal muscles help to protect the organs of respiration as well as contribute to their function. The bones of the thorax – the ribs, sternum and thoracic vertebrae – together with the diaphragm and intercostal muscles are responsible for effective breathing. Stress is associated with shallow or **apical** breathing whilst relaxation is associated with deep **diaphragmatic** breathing. Normal or **lateral costal** breathing constitutes the majority of our breathing and periods of stressful apical breathing, e.g. during intense or excessive physical activity, should be counteracted with periods of relaxing diaphragmatic breathing.

Water

Bones contain approximately 25 per cent water and muscles approximately 75 per cent. Lack of water leads to dry, brittle bones, stiff joints and a loss of muscle strength, power and speed. As a result the skeletal/muscular systems become vulnerable to attack and damage. Water is therefore vital for the well-being of these systems and should be consumed on a regular basis throughout the day increasing the amounts before, during and after increased activity.

- Drinking water prior to strenuous activity and exercise prevents dehydration.
- Drinking water during any activity and exercise in particular maintains fluid levels within the body, allowing water to be lost through sweating in order to control body temperature.
- Drinking water after strenuous activity and exercise helps to flush out the waste products produced in the skeletal/muscular systems as a result of energy production.

Nutrition

Foods vital for maintaining the functions of the skeletal/muscular systems include carbohydrates, fats, minerals and vitamins.

Fascinating Fact

Dust is largely made up of skin cells shed from the human body!

Angel advice

Reflexology encourages us to become more aware of our breathing. Breathing exercises should be given as part of the aftercare advice to enhance the effects of the treatment.

Angel advice

It is possible to drink too much water. If you drink at least 5 litres over too short a space of time you will get water intoxication. The sodium levels in the blood become diluted making the cells swell which in turn can cause nausea, headaches, confusion and in very rare situations, coma.

Fascinating Fact

Muscle cramps are often caused by calcium and magnesium imbalance within the body.

Fascinating Fact

A deficiency in manganese contributes to childhood growing pains and general pain in joints.

Fascinating Fact

Vital nutrients may be prevented from being absorbed into the body by smoking, alcohol, pollution, stress, fried foods etc.

- Carbohydrates for energy. Glycogen is the end product of carbohydrates and is stored within muscle fibres by the mitochondria. Excess glycogen is stored in the liver to be used by the muscles when their store has been depleted.
- Fats provide a back up energy source. A certain amount of fat is stored in yellow bone marrow. Fat is also stored as adipose tissue which forms the lower layer of the skin (hypodermis or subcutaneous layer) protecting the underlying muscles and bones.
- Calcium for bone density and effective muscle contractions.
- Magnesium for strong bones and healthy muscles.
- Manganese for the formation of healthy bones and cartilage.
- Sodium is needed for voluntary and involuntary muscle contractions.
- Zinc aids in the formation of bones.
- Vitamins A, C and E to combat the effects of free radicals.
- Vitamin D assists in maintaining strong and healthy bones by retaining calcium.

Remember

Free radicals are the toxic by-products of energy metabolism which contribute to premature ageing of the body.

Ageing

Babies are born with soft bones which gradually harden with age, reaching maturity when a person reaches the age of 25. Muscles change shape as a person reaches puberty developing into the male and female characteristics. Hormones are responsible for informing bones when to stop growing and muscles when to develop. As we age further, reaching menopause in women and andropause in men and the secretion of sex hormones lessens, there is a gradual reduction in the efficiency of the skeletal/muscular systems to perform their vital functions. Bones decrease in strength, joints lose their flexibility and muscles atrophy and weaken. The skeleton appears to shrink and lines, wrinkles and dropped contours develop as the skeletal muscles are less able to resist the pull of gravity. Free radical damage adds to the degenerative process associated with ageing as individual bone and muscle cells gradually lose their ability to take in nutrients and release waste products. This gradual deterioration has the effect of increasing the body's vulnerability to stress.

Fascinating Fact

The medical profession are beginning to recognise that a male goes through changes similar to those experienced in females during menopause. The name given to this stage in a male's life is andropause, signifying a pause or change in the secretion of androgens (male sex hormones).

Remember

Reflexology treatment provides the ideal opportunity for a person to rest their body and allow their own internal healing mechanisms to be activated.

Angel advice

As you are beginning to discover, the body craves balance in all things!

Tip

Improving coordination through activity effectively exercises the links between the skeletal/muscular and nervous systems, helping to improve both brain and muscle power!

Rest

If the skeletal/muscular systems are stressed and imbalanced, they need time to rest.

Rest ensures that any oxygen debt that has built up during excessive activity is repaid, allowing time for aching muscles to rid themselves of the waste products associated with energy production e.g. lactic acid. Rest also encourages the relaxation of muscles and joints, reducing the amount of muscle fibres contracting at any one time thus reducing the build up of muscular tension.

Although rest provides many rejuvenating and regenerating benefits to the skeletal/muscular systems, excessive rest can have a detrimental effect, as muscle and bone mass is lost during long periods of inactivity.

Activity

The skeletal/muscular systems naturally develop greater strength during periods of activity.

- Bones will build up their store of minerals when needed to perform increased activity over a period of time making them more durable and resilient.
- Muscles will build up their levels of power, strength, speed, endurance and flexibility through increased use, making them more efficient and effective.

Varied activity is of prime importance to the skeletal/muscular systems enabling the bones, joints and muscles to engage in a range of movements that are challenging both physically and psychologically, thus helping to maintain the function and form of the body as a whole.

Awareness

Throughout the day the skeletal/muscular systems are called upon to perform many functions – it takes 72 different muscles just to speak, and 200 to walk! This activity is coordinated by the brain and activated through the production of energy from nutrients received by the respiratory (oxygen) and digestive systems (food) via the circulatory system. It is therefore important to be aware of the additional benefits to the whole body when applying relaxation and pressure movements during a reflexology treatment to the skeletal/muscular systems. Of equal importance is to have an awareness of the factors that would prevent or restrict (contraindicate) the treatment and those age-related factors that would help to determine the depth of pressure. Care should be taken when treating babies, children and young adults as their bones and muscles are still forming, and with the elderly who may be experiencing bone and muscle weakness as a result of the ageing process.

Angel advice

When sitting at a computer or in the car a person's eyes should have a central view when the head is in the correct position. If this is not the case, the height of the chair should be altered accordingly.

Angel advice

As a person becomes more stressed and tense the shoulders automatically tighten and rise.

Remember

Heavy bags and children carried on one side of the body alters alignment, causing excess stress in corresponding muscles.

Tip

High heeled shoes will cause the knees to lock in an attempt to maintain balance, putting excessive strain on the knee and ankle joints. This is often felt as hard skin develops on corresponding reflexes on the feet, hands and ears as the body's way of trying to protect itself.

Special care

Stress manifests itself in a variety of ways and the skeletal/muscular systems are amongst the first systems to suffer. Symptoms including aching muscles and stiff joints accompany periods of excessive stress, creating an imbalance that affects body alignment and posture. Poor posture in turn creates a domino effect in other body systems, placing a massive strain on well-being. The reflexology treatment picks up on the effects of such strain, highlighting troubled areas. As a result care should be taken to ensure correct posture is maintained to avoid conditions associated with continuous use of individual muscles e.g. frozen shoulder, repetitive strain injury (**RSI**) etc.

Correcting posture involves careful analysis of the skeletal/muscular systems with subsequent corrective exercise advice.

Correct posture involves:

- Head held with the chin parallel to the floor when looking ahead to avoid undue neck strain. Care should be taken to return the head to this position after movement.
- Shoulders should be level and even i.e. scapula bones at equal distance from the spine, equal tone in pectoral and trapezium muscles avoiding shoulders rounding either forwards or backwards.
- Maintenance of natural curvature of the spine at each juncture i.e. cervical, thoracic, lumbar, sacral and coccyx curves.
- Balance in muscle tone between the rectus abdominus and errector spinae and gluteal muscles of the abdomen, back and buttocks helping to keep both the tummy and the bottom in.
- Balance in tone between the oblique muscles of the waist.
- Soft knees that do not over extend creating loss of balance and alignment.
- Equal body weight placed on both feet.

There are many benefits in maintaining correct posture including:

- Full and deep breathing can take place as the lungs are able to inflate with air without restriction.
- Digestive functions are improved as the organs tend to become compressed when posture is poor contributing to digestive problems e.g. indigestion etc.
- Postural problems e.g. kyphosis, lordosis and scoliosis area avoided due to the even distribution of body weight.
- Improved body image and confidence as a more flattering effect to the body is achieved making clothes look and feel better.

Case study

Most clients seeking reflexology treatment complain of stress and are experiencing stress-related symptoms associated with the skeletal/muscular system, usually in the form of tired, aching muscles and loss of free movement in joints such as the neck and shoulders.

It is always useful to start to work over the reflexes for these systems directly after the relaxation techniques are completed.

- Working the head reflex stimulates blood flow to the brain, helping to clear the mind and rationalise thoughts. This in turn helps to progress the therapeutic benefits gained from the massage movements associated with the relaxation techniques used post-consultation.

- Working the spinal reflexes eases out the tension in the corresponding muscles, in particular the erector spinae and trapezius muscles, and clients often experience a clicking and/or a tingling sensation as the vertebrae seem to ease their way back into place and the neuromuscular pathways begin to clear. Nerve responses and blood flow to and from the brain is automatically improved and brain activity is enhanced due to nerve responses travelling more freely along the spinal cord to and from the brain.

- Working the thorax reflex helps to ease out the chest area, which is often tight and compressed when a person is stressed. Such release facilitates deeper breathing and it is at this point that a client often automatically takes a deep breath as they begin to really relax into the treatment.

- Working the joint reflexes continues to ease out the tension and helps to create a greater flow of fluid within the synovial capsules surrounding the joints. Clients will often experience greater ease of movement as a result of working these reflexes.

Angel advice

The individual joints are more easily located on the ears due to the mirror image effect associated with the inverted foetus theory.

Angel advice

There is no set order of work in reflexology as long as relaxation movements start and end the treatment. The order of working the reflexes is up to the practitioner and should reflect the needs of the client.

Working the musculoskeletal system has a therapeutic effect on the whole body, releasing tense muscles and allowing greater ease of movement in joints, freeing neuromuscular pathways and encouraging total relaxation. Breathing becomes deeper and the body becomes energised and revitalised as a result of increased oxygen levels. Circulation is stimulated and immunity is improved. For this reason it makes sense to start working the reflexes with this system, although they may be worked at any point throughout the treatment.

Self-help can form a large part of the aftercare for the skeletal/muscular system by encouraging the client to work the skeletal/muscular reflexes on their own hands. Just as the neck benefits from being massaged and rubbed so do the corresponding reflex points, and such advice can be given without fear of misuse or ill effect.

Task

Using the treatment card as a guide work over the skeletal/muscular reflexes on the feet, hands or ears. Mark down on the card when an area comes up. It may be that the client is alerted to the reflex by experiencing a tingling sensation, a slight pain or general discomfort in the form of tenderness etc. In addition, you may feel a tightness, puffiness, grittiness etc. in the corresponding area. Note this down by placing a mark in the corresponding box. You may want to tick or cross the box or even shade it in. By shading it in, you can shade part or the entire box to reflect what was felt. Start with a consultation and continue with relaxation movements. After working the reflexes finish with further relaxation movements, breathing exercises, feedback and relevant aftercare advice.

Knowledge review

1   What is the approximate percentage of water in bones and muscles?

2   What is the function of red bone marrow?

3   Name the three types of joints.

4   What are the functions of ligaments and tendons?

5   Give four functions of the skeletal/muscular systems.

6   What does the abbreviation RSI stand for?

7   Name the five regions of the spine.

8   Where on the feet are the spinal reflexes found?

9   Where is the reflex point for the shoulder located on the hands?

10   In which part of the ear are the reflexes for the joints located?

15

Reflexes of the respiratory system

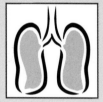

The respiratory system can be divided up into two main parts – the upper and lower respiratory tracts. The upper respiratory tract consists of the **nose, sinuses, pharynx** and **larynx**; the lower respiratory tract consists of the **trachea, bronchi** and **lungs**:

Upper respiratory tract

- The nose – providing the main point of entry for air coming into the body and the main point of exit for air leaving the body. The nostrils form two separate openings into the nasal cavity which is lined with ciliated mucous membrane forming layers of hair-like cells called cilia, which filter air as it enters. Mucus is produced by goblet cells and is thick and slimy, trapping any minute particles in the air as it enters the nose.

Fascinating Fact

Particles picked up in the nose initiate the sneeze reflex ensuring exit out of the body!

- Sinuses – air spaces in the bones of the skull i.e. frontal, ethmoid, sphenoid and maxillae bones, all of which open onto the nasal cavity. These sinuses are lined with epithelial tissue containing goblet cells that secrete mucus.
- Pharynx – the back of the throat leading on from the nasal cavity. It is divided into three sections – naso, oro and laryngo. The nasopharynx contains the **Eustachian tube**, linking the nasal cavity with the ears. The oropharynx provides a passageway for food and air entering the body via

Fascinating Fact

Lacrimal glands or tear glands are situated in recesses in the frontal bones. They secrete fluid in the form of tears which leave the glands by small ducts passing over the front of the eyes under the lids where they drain into the nasal cavity through a small canal.

the mouth and the laryngopharynx provides the passageway for food to enter the oesophagus. The adenoids and tonsils are located within the naso and oropharynx respectively.

Remember

Adenoids and tonsils consist of lymphatic tissue and contribute to the immune functions of the body by filtering harmful substances from the air.

- Larynx – leading on from the pharynx, the larynx forms the upper throat and contains the vocal cords. The larynx also contains a lid-like structure called the epiglottis which prevents food from entering the lower respiratory tract when we swallow.

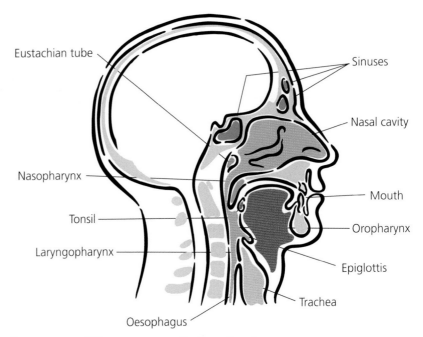

Structures of the upper respiratory tract

Lower respiratory tract

- Trachea – leading on from the larynx, the trachea is commonly known as the windpipe. It forms a semi-solid passageway for air.
- Bronchi – the trachea divides into smaller passageways forming the left and right bronchi which lead into each lung.

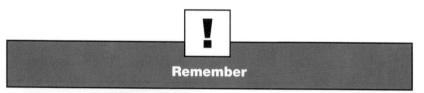

Remember

Filtering of the incoming air continues into the lower respiratory tract by the trachea and bronchi. Any trapped particles initiate the cough reflex.

Remember

The left lung is smaller than the right to allow room in the chest for the heart.

- Lungs – soft, spongy balloon-like structures situated on either side of the heart. Within the lungs, the bronchi subdivide to form smaller tubes called bronchioles which end in tiny sac-like structures called alveoli where the exchange of gases e.g. oxygen and carbon dioxide takes place.

The bones and muscles of the thorax provide protection for the structures of the lower respiratory tract.

The respiratory system is responsible for respiration involving five individual processes: breathing, external respiration, transportation, internal respiration and cellular respiration.

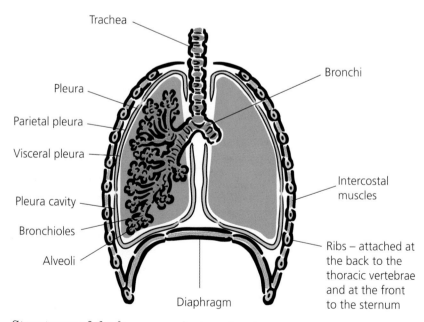

Structures of the lower respiratory tract

1. Breathing – can be defined as the movement of air in and out of the lungs by inspiration or inhalation and expiration or exhalation.

2. Internal respiration – the exchange of oxygen from the air with carbon dioxide in the blood takes place within the alveoli in the lungs.

3. Transportation – the pulmonary circulation ensures that oxygen is transported to the heart (via pulmonary veins) for distribution around the body and that carbon dioxide is transported from the heart (via pulmonary arteries) to the lungs for exit out of the body.

Remember

The heart is made from cardiac muscular tissue and acts like a pump. It is the centre of the blood circulatory system and is involved with the transportation of blood to and from all parts of the body.

4. Internal respiration – oxygenated blood from the heart and lungs is received by the cells of the body where it is replaced with carbon dioxide. Deoxygenated blood is then transported back to the heart and lungs and the whole process repeated.

5. Cellular respiration – the utilisation of oxygen in the cells and the production of carbon dioxide. The individual cells use the oxygen to form energy and as a result produce carbon dioxide.

It is important to appreciate that every living cell is dependent on the act of breathing for survival, and care should be taken to ensure that the rate and depth of breathing matches the needs of the body. Although this is controlled by the autonomic nervous system, everyday factors such as stress and poor posture can put excessive strain on the respiratory system resulting in inadequate breathing techniques. This in turn affects the performance of the cells, tissues, organs and systems of the body. Reflexology can help to balance the activity within the system, aiding the well-being of the body as a whole.

 Fascinating Fact

The **solar plexus** provides the link between the autonomic nervous system and the respiratory systems through a set of nerves which stimulate the lungs in response to stress. Solar refers to the sun and the effects of this plexus radiate like the sun's rays.

System sorter

RESPIRATORY SYSTEM

Nervous system

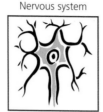

The nervous system is alerted when tiny particles have been trapped by the ciliated mucous membrane lining the respiratory tracts and activates the sneeze and cough reflexes. The nervous system is also able to determine the body's need for oxygen and activates the diaphragm to contract, ensuring that breathing takes place.

Circulatory system

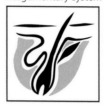

Blood transports the oxygen breathed into the lungs all around the body for use by each living cell. As a result, carbon dioxide is produced and is transported by the blood to the lungs to be released out of the body as we breathe out.

Integumentary system

The skin, hair and nails rely on the oxygen breathed into the lungs and transported by the blood for the constant renewal of cells. A good supply of oxygen together with a good blood supply ensures healthy skin, hair and nails.

Skeletal/muscular systems

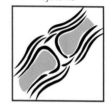

The bones of the thorax – 12 thoracic vertebrae, 12 pairs of ribs and the sternum – offer protection to the heart and lungs. The intercostal muscles and the diaphragm help in the process of breathing by contracting to enlarge the space to let maximum air into the lungs.

Immune system

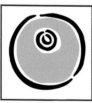

The adenoids, situated in the nasopharynx, and the tonsils, situated in the oropharynx, are comprised of lymphatic tissue which helps to contribute to the immune functions of the respiratory system by filtering harmful substances from the air.

Parts of the respiratory system like the nose, throat and windpipe contain ciliated columnar cells which form an epithelial lining or ciliated mucous membrane. The purpose of these cells is to trap unwanted particles, preventing them from entering the lungs and causing damage to the body.

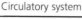

Cells

The kidneys compensate for water lost from the body through breathing by monitoring fluid levels within the body and holding onto water when necessary. As a result urine becomes more concentrated.

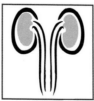

Genito-urinary system

The adrenal glands secrete the hormone adrenalin in response to a stressful situation, which in turn has the effect of increasing breathing rate. When the stressful situation has passed, adrenalin secretion subsides and breathing returns to normal.

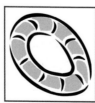

Endocrine system

The lymphatic system is responsible for draining and filtering excess fluid and waste from the respiratory system, contributing to the immune functions of this system. Drainage of lymph from the thoracic and right lymphatic ducts into the subclavian veins takes place in the thoracic region of the body.

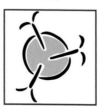

Lymphatic system

The oropharynx forms the link between the digestive and respiratory systems. Muscular coordination in the larynx separates the systems, with the action of the epiglottis blocking off entry into the trachea during swallowing.

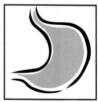

Digestive system

Consultation considerations

In order to determine the levels of stress imposed upon the respiratory systems and its contributory systems i.e. circulation, it may be necessary to take note of the following considerations during the consultation process:

Oral

As well as asking about major respiratory conditions e.g. asthma etc. and associated medication it is also useful to ask the client about the type and frequency of common complaints – common cold, sinusitis, ear infections etc. – affecting the respiratory system. This will give an indication of the strength of the immune system in fighting off common ailments and, as immunity is lowered through stress, it will also give an indication of stress levels and a person's ability to cope. It is also useful to ascertain whether or not the client smokes, either in the past or at present, and whether actively or passively.

Tip

A useful question to ask is "How often do you suffer with a cold and which areas does it tend to affect?" The answers given will lead to other questions which will in turn lead to a greater understanding of the person as a whole.

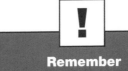

Remember

As the blood circulatory system is so closely linked with the respiratory system it is also useful to ask about conditions affecting the heart – high or low blood pressure etc. and associated medication, as it may be necessary to seek medical advice prior to carrying out a reflexology treatment.

Visual

It is important to observe the client's rate and depth of breathing and whether or not it changes during the consultation. This will provide an insight into their physical, physiological and psychological well-being – depth of breathing is often associated with posture, exertion and nervousness, frustration etc. and rate of breathing is often associated with exertion levels, heart and lung problems, fear, anger etc. The results of such observation will determine a person's stress levels and once again demonstrate their ability to cope.

Links between the respiratory, circulatory and nervous systems may be seen in the colour of the skin, which will provide an indication of the condition of their blood circulation and associated levels of sensitivity e.g. high colouring denotes blood vessels that may be close to the surface and more sensitive to touch. Colour also provides an external sign to a person's inner feelings e.g. a red complexion indicates anger or embarrassment, whilst a white, pale complexion indicates someone who may be drained of emotion etc.

Aural

Listening to the way in which a client uses their breathing is a useful tool in the consultation process. Efficient breathing allows for the production of sound through the vocal cords situated in the larynx. Speech occurs during expiration (outward breath) when the tongue, cheeks and lips manipulate the sounds produced by the vocal cords. Inefficient breathing results in poor quality of sound, pitch and tone. In addition, nervousness may result in stammering or the inability to find the right words.

Olfactory

The smell of cigarette smoke may alert the practitioner to the fact that the client is either a smoker or has been subjected to cigarette smoke in their immediate environment. These facts are necessary in determining the possible damaging effect to the respiratory system and associated systems e.g. circulatory, as well as providing a starting point for aftercare advice in terms of suggested avoidance techniques.

 Angel advice

Smoking cigarettes has an effect on both the respiratory and circulatory systems affecting the intake, transportation and utilisation of oxygen by the cells of the body.

Perceptive

Breathing provides a link between people as one person's breath out constitutes a part of another person's breath in. The invisible barrier that is formed between people takes this intimacy into consideration, as we tend to avoid close contact with strangers. However, it may be possible to pick up on the way in which a person is feeling about themselves and the world around them by the way in which they are breathing. Shallow breathing is often associated with feelings of low self-esteem, as a person feels unworthy of forming a deep connection with their surroundings and the people within it.

Tactile

Conducting the relaxation movements post-consultation provides a means for further investigation through touch. Touching the areas generally associated with the respiratory system together with the specific respiratory reflexes on the feet, hands or ears will help to determine the possible stresses and strains. The areas associated with the nose, sinuses, throat and lungs etc. commonly feel tight, puffy and/or congested in much the same way as the areas themselves. When touching a person's feet, hands or ears you are in effect picking up externally on the feelings that they themselves are experiencing internally. These movements also stimulate blood circulation, generally helping to benefit the whole of the body.

Contraindication considerations

It is important to avoid treating a client suffering with severe respiratory problems and those of its associated system of circulation without medical approval. These combined systems contribute to the well-being of the body as a whole throughout life through breathing and the transportation of oxygen and carbon dioxide in the blood. It is therefore important that medical supervision is also sought in the event of medical approval being given to ensure that the treatment remains complementary.

 Angel advice

Disorders such as ACROCYANOSIS – deficiency in the circulation of the hands and feet – and RAYNAUD'S SYNDROME – contraction of the arteries supplying blood to the hands and feet causing numbness – need extreme care and may indicate treatment of the ears (if unaffected) as an alternative to the feet and hands.

Reflexes

Pressure movements performed generally, e.g. along the longitudinal and/or transverse zones of the feet and hands, will produce a general affect on the respiratory system and have a knock-on effect on the circulatory system as well as the other systems of the body. Working the specific reflexes will help the well-being of these isolated areas, contributing to the well-being of the system and so the body as a whole.

Remember

The nasopharynx contains the adenoids, the oropharnyx contains the tonsils and the larynx contains the vocal cords.

Remember

The solar plexus is a network of nerves lying just below the diaphragm and is often referred to as the great sympathetic plexus.

The position of the reflexes

The reflexes for the respiratory system lie in the upper section of the feet/hands between the diaphragm line and the tip of the toes/fingers and the lower section of the ears.

- Nose – contained within the dorsal aspect of the big toe and thumb (face) and the centre of the junction between the ear lobe and the cheek.
- Throat (pharynx and larynx) – the lateral base of the big toe, thumb and where the base of the helix meets the top part of the ear canal.
- Ears – along the base of the fourth and fifth toes/fingers and the border separating the outer and inner surface of the tragus on the ear.
- Eustachian tube – the gap between the base of the third and fourth toes/fingers. No specific reflex on the ear.
- Eyes – along the base of the second and third toes/fingers and the centre of the lobe of the ear.
- Sinuses – the plantar aspect of the four small toes and the palmar aspect of the fingers. There is no specific reflex point on the ears but the sinuses are worked when working corresponding areas.
- Mouth – the dorsal aspect of the small toes/fingers and the base of the helix.
- Trachea/bronchi – from base of the big toe/thumb to the diaphragm line and lower concha of the ear.
- Lungs – between the shoulder line and diaphragm line in zones 2 – 4 of the feet/hands and the centre of the lower concha of the ear.
- Heart – situated predominantly on the left foot/hand above the diaphragm line and in the lower concha of the ear.
- Solar plexus – slightly off centre on the diaphragm line towards the medial edge on the feet/hands. There is no specific reflex point for the solar plexus on the ears. However, the point zero acts on the respiratory system encouraging deep, calm breathing.

 Fascinating Fact

The reflex point known as point zero links the nervous and endocrine systems and is the central point of the ear. Working this point relieves stress generally.

Respiratory system – order of work

The adenoids and tonsils will be affected by working the throat reflex.

The ears have three main functions – hearing, balance and maintenance of pressure.

The jaw is made up of the upper maxillae and lower mandible bones containing the gums and the teeth. Also contained within the mouth are the hard and soft palates, the tongue and the salivary glands. Any tension felt in this area may relate to any of these areas as well as the muscles responsible for jaw movements.

The heart is situated on the left side of the chest and as such is located mainly on the left foot.

Suggested order of work – feet

The head and face are treated generally on the whole of the big toe, incorporating all of the upper respiratory system, blood and lymphatic vessels and nerves. Order of work for specific reflexes include:

The upper respiratory tract

The throat and sinus reflexes and the contributory reflexes of the ears, eyes and mouth (jaw).

- *Throat* – using the index finger hook in and back up into the base of the lateral aspect (outer side towards the second toe) of the big toe. Press three times.
- *Ears* – using the thumb or index finger work along the ridge at the base of the plantar aspect of the toes, starting at the little toe and working towards the next toe.
- *Eustachian tube* – pivot on the point between the base of the fourth and third toes.
- *Eyes* – proceed along the ridge at the base of the toes. The next two toes represent the eye.
- *Sinuses* – work up the plantar aspect (underside) of the four small toes. Use a soothing movement to drain.
- *Jaw* – using the index finger work down the dorsal aspect (top) of each of the four small toes from the base of each nail to the base of each toe. The fourth and fifth toes relate to the lower jaw and the second and third toes to the upper jaw.

The lower respiratory tract

The trachea, bronchi and lung reflexes and the contributory reflexes of the heart and solar plexus.

- *Trachea/bronchi* – using the thumb or index finger work down from the centre of the big toe (plantar surface) towards the diaphragm line. Repeat three times.
- *Lungs/heart* – work transversely, diagonally or longitudinally along zones 1–5 of the plantar surface of the feet from the shoulder line (base of toes) to the diaphragm line. This will work the lungs, heart and surrounding areas i.e. muscles, blood and lymph vessels and nerves. By overlapping the rows and working with alternate thumbs/fingers from zone 1 to zone 5 and back from zone 5 to zone 1 you will ensure adequate coverage of the whole area.
- *Solar plexus* – place the thumb pad slightly off centre of the diaphragm line facing towards the medial arch. Gently pivot on the point.

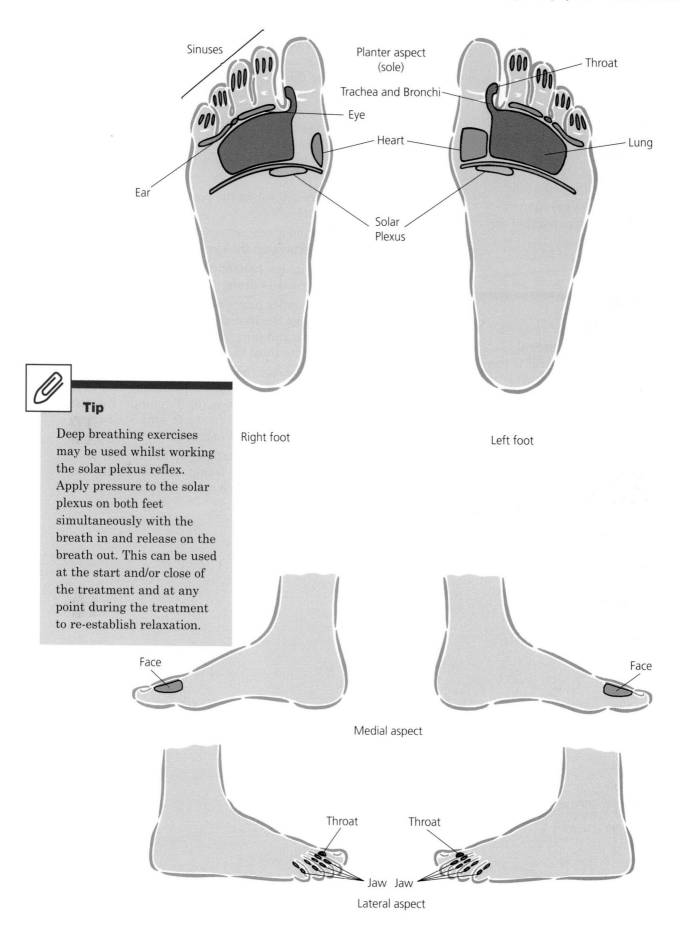

Sinuses

Planter aspect
(sole)

Throat

Trachea and Bronchi

Eye

Heart

Lung

Ear

Solar
Plexus

Right foot

Left foot

Tip

Deep breathing exercises
may be used whilst working
the solar plexus reflex.
Apply pressure to the solar
plexus on both feet
simultaneously with the
breath in and release on the
breath out. This can be used
at the start and/or close of
the treatment and at any
point during the treatment
to re-establish relaxation.

Face

Face

Medial aspect

Throat   Throat

Jaw Jaw

Lateral aspect

Suggested order of work – hands

- *Throat* – using the index finger hook in and back up into the base of the lateral aspect of the thumb. Press three times.
- *Ears* – using the thumb or index finger work along the ridge at the base of the palmar aspect of the fingers, starting at the little finger and working towards the next finger.
- *Eustachian tube* – pivot on the point between the fourth and third fingers.
- *Eyes* – proceed along the base of the fingers. The third and second fingers represent the eye.
- *Sinuses* – work up the palmar aspect of all four fingers. Use soothing movements to drain.
- *Jaw* – using the index finger work down the dorsal aspect of each finger from the base of each nail to the base of each finger. The fourth and fifth fingers relate to the lower jaw and the second and third to the upper jaw.
- *Trachea / bronchi / lungs / heart* – work transversely, diagonally or longitudinally on the palmar surface of the hands from the shoulder line to the diaphragm line using small overlapping rows from zone 1 to zone 5. Change hands and work from zone 5 to zone 1.
- *Solar plexus* – place the thumb pad in the slightly off centre of the diaphragm line facing towards the medial edge of the hand. Gently pivot on the point.

Tip

Working the sinus reflexes on the hands is often more effective than working the feet.

Tip

The representation of organs in the hands is more compressed than that of the feet and it is more difficult to isolate some structures e.g. trachea/bronchi. Working the shoulder to diaphragm line ensures all areas are worked.

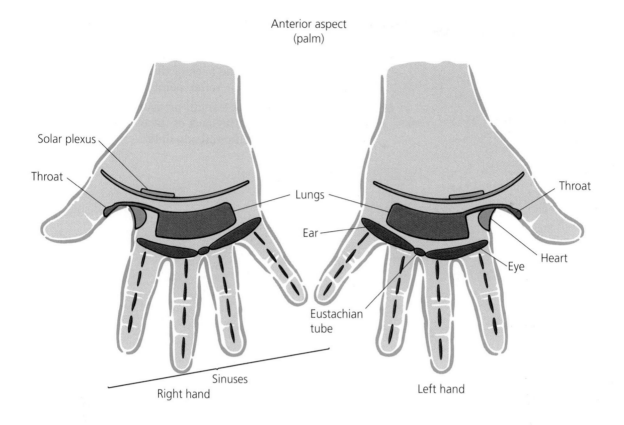

Anterior aspect
(palm)

Solar plexus

Throat

Lungs

Ear

Throat

Heart

Eye

Eustachian
tube

Sinuses

Right hand

Left hand

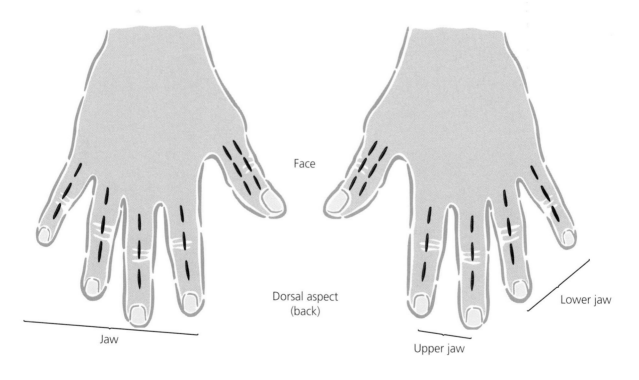

Face

Dorsal aspect
(back)

Jaw

Upper jaw

Lower jaw

Tip

Point zero may be used in the same way as the solar plexus to encourage deep breathing and establish relaxation.

Suggested order of work – ears

- *Upper respiratory tract* – small pressure movements using the thumb to support the back of the ear and index finger to work over the specific reflex points.
- *Lower respiratory tract* – small pressure movements using the thumb to support the back of the ear and index finger to work over the specific reflex points.

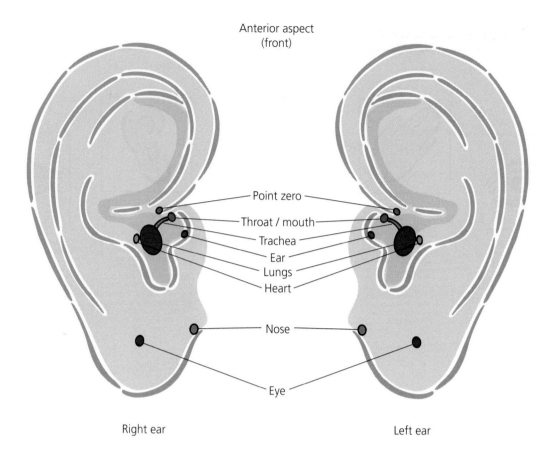

Anterior aspect
(front)

Point zero
Throat / mouth
Trachea
Ear
Lungs
Heart

Nose

Eye

Right ear

Left ear

Treatment tracker

RESPIRATORY SYSTEM

Visualisation

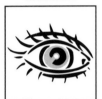

Rising stress levels increase the breathing rate; visualisations that relax the mind in turn relax the body. Try to visualise your body slowly opening itself up, like a flower unfolding in the gentle warmth of the sun. Watch how each petal unfurls itself tentatively revealing first the tip, then the centre and finally the whole of itself. Visualise the warm air surrounding the flower becoming a part of its whole being as it permeates every part of every petal until it has reached the very core. Now focus on your own body feeling the openness as your breathing has become more relaxed, deeper and freer. Regular use of visualisation techniques helps to counteract the effects of stress as well as help to prepare the body for deeper relaxation techniques e.g. meditation.

Hands

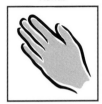

The respiratory system is located in the upper part of the hands on both the dorsal and palmar aspects. Working the upper parts of the respiratory system on the hands provides easier access to the reflexes associated with the sinuses and the mouth/jaw in particular because of their position on the fingers. This provides an excellent site for self-treatment.

Feet

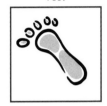

The respiratory system is located in the upper part of the feet on both the dorsal and plantar aspects. Treating the respiratory system on the feet provides a means for total relaxation which in turn improves the system's vital functions associated with respiration. Incorporating breathing exercises whilst treating the respiratory system increases the effectiveness of the treatment.

Ears

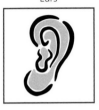

The respiratory system lies within the lower concha of the ear. Point zero, situated in the centre of the ear, provides a reflex point which has an immediate calming influence on the body, helping to regulate breathing. This reflex point provides a useful site for self-treatment and has been used with success to aid addictive behaviour and help to alleviate fear and extreme nervousness.

Affirmation

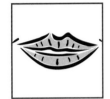

Effective breathing takes time and all too often we find ourselves and our breathing speeding up. Affirmations can be used to slow breathing down, calm the body, and energise the mind. Check your posture and concentrate on your breathing. When you have your breathing under control try to imagine the word 'my' as you breath deeply in through the nose. As you breathe out open your mouth and say the word 'time' out loud releasing maximum amounts of air as you get to the end of the word. Repeat three or four times whenever you feel stress levels are increasing out of control. You are using 'your time' for the benefit of your body!

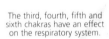
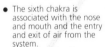

The third, fourth, fifth and sixth chakras have an effect on the respiratory system.

- The sixth chakra is associated with the nose and mouth and the entry and exit of air from the system.
- The fifth chakra is associated with the pharynx, larynx, bronchi, bronchioles and upper lobes of the lungs and the functions of communication.
- The fourth chakra is associated with the lower section of the thorax, lower lobes of the lungs, the heart and the functions of transportation.
- The third chakra is associated with the autonomic nervous system and the functions of regulation.

Balancing the energy in these chakras benefits the physical and psychological aspects of their associated functions.

The colours white and blue are linked to the respiratory system. Their use is both calming and balancing, reducing sensitivity on a physical and psychological level. This helps to control the breathing rate and slow down the action of the heart. White and blue also have an anti-inflammatory effect which is useful for any respiratory problems. In addition, yellow is the colour associated with the solar plexus and has a stimulating affect on breathing, helping to improve the depth and flow. Although breathing is a natural skill it is also underused and breathing exercises before, during and after a reflexology treatment help to reinforce the benefits of good breath work.

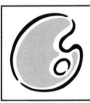

Colour

The respiratory system is located in all five longitudinal zones as well as the upper transverse zone. Treating these zones generally helps to free the energy, which in turn has a knock-on effect on the specific organs as well as those located in other parts of the zones e.g. treating the lungs in zones 2–4 will have an effect on all of the other organs located in zones 2–4. A problem associated with a specific organ often manifests itself with problems in the rest of the corresponding zone.

The lung meridian starts at the clavicle and ends at the back of the thumb. It is naturally stimulated from 3 a.m.–5 a.m. and naturally sedated from 3 p.m.–5 p.m. The yin lung meridian is coupled with the yang large intestine meridian and their problems may often be linked e.g. chest infection and constipation. Reflexology has an effect on the energy flow within the meridians, creating the potential for improved well-being. Because the energy flow through the meridians is continuous without beginning or end, the effects will be seen throughout the whole of the meridian system and the whole body.

The note G is associated with the respiratory system. Music that is rich in high tones and meditative music have a stimulating effect on the respiratory system. During reflexology the note G may be imagined or sung out loud whilst working over the respiratory system. The vibrations made by the sound will have an affect on the vibrations of the respiratory organs helping to balance and normalise their activity. If music is used, the body organs will pick up and respond to the individual notes, naturally creating a sense of harmony that is reflected in the well-being of the client, the practitioner and indeed the treatment room.

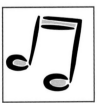

Sound

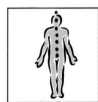

Chakras

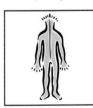

Zones

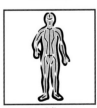

Meridians

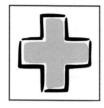

Common conditions

When treating problems associated with the respiratory system it is always advisable to complete a full treatment to include all reflexes, paying particular attention to those directly affecting the problem as well as those indirectly involved.

As stress is often the cause and/or a contributory factor in most problems affecting these systems, attention should be paid to the pituitary and adrenal glands for their role in the body's response to stress. The solar plexus reflex will need extra attention due to its de-stressing function. Particular attention should also be paid to the elimination reflexes of the body e.g. lymphatic nodes and ducts (see the lymphatic system, Chapter 19), kidneys, ureters and bladder (see the genito-urinary system, Chapter 17) for their role in ridding the body of the waste products associated with stress. In addition, because of the fact that mucus from the respiratory system may be swallowed, attention should be paid throughout the treatment to the digestive system for its role in digestion and elimination. The list below gives common conditions together with their suggested direct and indirect reflexes.

An A–Z of common conditions affecting the respiratory system

Activity

Working through each condition, try to analyse the reasons for paying particular attention to the indirect reflexes. Refer to the reflexes for the appropriate body systems within this chapter for more information.

- ADENOID enlarged – can block the opening of the Eustachian tube and/or obstruct airflow from the nose to the throat. *Direct reflex* = Eustachian tube. *Indirect reflexes* = throat, face, sinuses.

- ASTHMA – difficulty in breathing caused by narrowing of the airways. It may be triggered off by external factors known as extrinsic asthma or internal factors known as intrinsic asthma. *Direct reflex* = the lungs. *Indirect reflexes* = heart, throat, sinuses, trachea, thorax and thoracic spine, shoulder.

- BRONCHITIS – inflammation of the lining of the bronchi. *Direct reflex* = the lungs. *Indirect reflexes* = heart, trachea, thorax and thoracic spine, shoulder.

- COMMON COLD – contagious viral infection resulting in a sore throat and runny nose. Usually lasts for 2–7 days with full recovery taking up to three weeks. *Direct reflex* = the most affected area e.g. the nose/face. *Indirect reflexes* = associated areas e.g. ears, sinuses, throat, eyes etc.

- COUGH – voluntary or reflex expulsion of air from the lungs to expel a foreign body or accumulation of mucus. *Direct reflex* = the lungs. *Indirect reflexes* = trachea, throat.

- CROUP – viral infection that affects children. Characterised by a hoarse, barking cough and a fever. *Direct reflex* = the throat. *Indirect reflexes* = trachea, lungs, thorax and thoracic spine, thymus gland.

- EMPHYSEMA – inflammation of the alveoli in the lungs causing blood flow through the lungs to slow down. It is usually associated with bronchitis and/or old age. *Direct reflex* = the lungs. *Indirect reflexes* = trachea, thorax and thoracic spine, cervical spine, neck.

- GLANDULAR FEVER – a viral infection, which is most common in the 15–22 year old age group. It is characterised by a persistent sore throat and/or tonsillitis. *Direct reflex* = the throat. *Indirect reflexes* = face, head, trachea, lungs, thorax and thoracic spine, thymus gland.

- HAY FEVER – caused by an allergy to pollen. Hay fever commonly affects the nose, eyes and sinuses as the pollen irritates these areas causing excessive sneezing, watery eyes and a build up of mucus. The airways may also be affected resulting in wheezing as breathing becomes more difficult. *Direct reflex* = affected area e.g. eyes, nose/face. *Indirect reflexes* = sinuses, throat, trachea, thorax and thoracic spine.

- HYPERVENTILATION – rapid deep breathing commonly associated with stress. *Direct reflex* = the lungs. *Indirect reflexes* = heart, thorax and thoracic spine, shoulders, head and face.

- LARYNGITIS – inflammation of the larynx producing hoarseness and/or loss of voice. There are two forms – acute, which develops quickly and is short lived and chronic, which is recurring. *Direct reflex* = the throat. *Indirect reflexes* = lungs, neck, shoulders, throat.

- LUNG CANCER – a life threatening, malignant growth (tumour) in the lungs. *Direct reflex* = the lungs. *Indirect reflexes* = trachea, throat, thorax and thoracic spine, thymus gland.

- NASAL POLYP – harmless extensions of the mucous lining within the nasal cavity containing fluid causing an obstruction in air flow. *Direct reflex* = face/nose. *Indirect reflexes* = Eustachian tube, throat.

- PHARYNGITIS – inflammation of the pharynx resulting in a sore throat which may be either acute or chronic. Acute pharyngitis is very common and clears up after a week or so. Chronic pharyngitis is longer lasting and can result from smoking. *Direct reflex* = the throat. *Indirect reflexes* = nose/face, Eustachian tube, ears.

- PLEURISY – inflammation of the pleura surrounding the lungs, usually occurs as a complication of other disorders. *Direct reflex* = the lungs. *Indirect reflexes* = trachea, thorax and thoracic spine.

- PNEUMONIA – inflammation of the lungs from either a bacterial or viral infection resulting in chest pain, dry cough, fever etc. Bacterial pneumonia tends to last longer. *Direct reflex* = lungs. *Indirect reflexes* = trachea, thorax and thoracic spine, spleen.

- RHINITIS – inflammation of the mucous lining of the nasal cavity causing a blocked, runny and stuffy nose. *Direct reflex* = nose/face. *Indirect reflexes* = eyes, ears, throat.

- SINUSITIS – inflammation of the mucous lining of the sinuses causing a blockage, which can be very painful, swollen and sore. It can be acute, usually accompanying a cold, or chronic when there are recurrent blockages. *Direct reflex* = the sinuses. *Indirect reflexes* = head, face, eyes, throat.
- STRESS – excessive stress causes the autonomic nervous system to activate the release of the hormone adrenalin. This causes the breathing rate to increase. *Direct reflexes* = the lungs. *Indirect reflexes* = heart, trachea, throat, shoulders, spine.
- TONSILLITIS – inflammation of the tonsils resulting in soreness in the throat generally. It is more common in children. *Direct reflex* = the throat. *Indirect reflexes* = Eustachian tube, ears, eyes, sinuses, neck, cervical spine, lungs.
- TUBERCULOSIS (TB) – infectious disease involving the formation of nodules in body tissue. The most common sites are the lungs. Immunisation is available. *Direct reflex* = the lungs. *Indirect reflexes* = trachea, throat, thyroid gland.

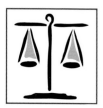

Holistic harmony

The respiratory system plays a vital role in keeping the body alive. It provides the entry point for oxygen, the life force of the body, and the exit point for unwanted carbon dioxide. Together with the circulatory system, the respiratory system services every cell, tissue organ and system and is responsible in part for every activity the body performs. Although designed for constant use these systems suffer with constant *misuse* and can only function to optimum levels with constant care. This can be achieved through regular reflexology treatment which helps to highlight the need for improved self-awareness, especially in terms of the following factors.

Air

Tip

Cigarette smoke contains small amounts of carbon monoxide.

The type of air breathed into the body will affect the functioning of the respiratory and circulatory systems and in turn the body as a whole. Pollution contributes to the type of air that is harmful to the body. Certain inhaled gases such as carbon monoxide make the transportation of oxygen difficult and although the body is capable of producing more red blood cells to help to counteract this effect, constant exposure to such gases has debilitating long-term effects.

As a result it is more efficient to breathe air into the body through the nose rather than the mouth because the air is:

- Filtered by the cilia inside the nasal cavity.
- Warmed by the blood in the nose adjusting the temperature of the air to that of the body.
- Moistened as water evaporates from the mucous lining.
- Smelt by the sensory nerves in the nose passing information to the brain which in turn identifies the smell.

Water

Breathing through the mouth results in a loss of small amounts of water from the body contributing to the drying out of the throat generally. Breathing through the nose helps to retain some of this water, making breathing more comfortable. Water also contributes to the distribution of oxygen and carbon dioxide around the body, which is much improved when the water content of the blood is high. Lack of water results in dehydration which may have the following effects:

- The volume of blood will fall resulting in reduced blood pressure and fainting.
- Blood thickens in the absence of water which can restrict flow and cause a rise in blood pressure.

Water is also needed for the formulation of tears, mucus and cerumen (earwax), all of which are needed for the protection of the respiratory system.

One-and-half litres a day of fresh, clean water in addition to a daily intake of fruit and vegetables will help to maintain the body's fluid levels.

Nutrition

A high intake of antioxidants such as Vitamins A, C, E and selenium are recommended to counteract the debilitating effects of free radicals and help to safeguard the body against cancer and heart disease.

Other useful nutrients include:

- Folic acid for the development of red blood cells.
- Iron for the development of haemoglobin in red blood cells.
- Vitamin B12 for the transportation of oxygen.
- Ginger to prevent blood clots.

Foods to avoid include:

- Mucus-forming foods, e.g. dairy products, which can irritate problems associated with the respiratory system. Such foods should be avoided when the problems are severe, and taken in moderation at other times especially if the problem is persistent and/or recurring.
- Saturated fats which contribute to furring of the arteries and poor transportation of oxygen.

Ageing

A baby uses its body intuitively and allows it to respond naturally. The young, uninhibited body works in a way that allows the respiratory system to function at optimum levels resulting in unrestricted breathing at all times. As we age we lose

Fascinating Fact

Lung cancer and heart attacks are amongst the biggest causes of death in the West and there is increasing evidence that the food we eat is a contributory factor.

Remember

Haemoglobin is a complex protein contained within red blood cells by which oxygen is transported.

Angel advice

Ginger is also very good for sore throats. To make a soothing ginger drink add boiling water to a few slices of root ginger. Add a cinnamon stick, lemon and honey to taste.

our intuitive skills, forcing unnatural conditions upon the body, sometimes pushing it to the limit whilst ignoring the many warning signs. Breathing is one of the skills that is forced into unnatural performance as we expose the body to excessive amounts of stress. Ageing is also responsible for a gradual slowing down of natural processes, putting additional strain on the systems if stress levels are high resulting in breathlessness and raised blood pressure.

Rest

Rest is associated with relaxation and a general slowing down of activity. This in turn leads to a slowing down in breathing and provides the opportunity to counteract the periods of increased breathing rate associated with stressful situations. The rate of breathing is controlled by the autonomic nervous system which also helps to activate the fight or flight response associated with stress, diverting blood to the muscles and away from the digestive system etc. Times of rest allow for the maintenance of homeostasis, keeping the body healthy, happy and balanced. Treating the solar plexus reflex during treatment helps to calm the autonomic nervous system responses reducing stress levels and returning breathing to normal.

The natural pull of gravity has an effect on venous blood flow and periods of rest with the feet and legs raised help the general free flow of deoxygenated blood back to the heart so that the carbon dioxide can then be released during exhalation.

Activity

Varied activity is vital for the well-being of the respiratory system and its contributory systems:

- Activity that promotes improved posture will have a direct result on improved breathing.
- Activity that strengthens the muscles associated with breathing, i.e. the intercostals and the diaphragm, allows breathing to become more efficient.
- Activity that increases the heart rate is beneficial in strengthening the lungs thus increasing their capacity for air.

Awareness

Having awareness of the links between the different parts of the respiratory system and those between other systems is a necessary ingredient for maintaining good health.

Ill health occurs when we ignore these links by misusing parts of the body that in turn affect the rest of the body finally resulting in illness. Although there are certain parts of the body we can live without i.e. an arm, a foot, the appendix, tonsils etc. the body relies on harmony between its vital parts to achieve and maintain homeostasis.

Angel advice

Venous blood supply relies on muscular activity to aid the flow of deoxygenated blood back to the heart.

Holistic treatments such as reflexology help to create awareness, highlighting and linking stressed areas of the body with signs and symptoms and also provide a means to rebalance and eventually maintain a general state of balance.

Angel advice

Thermal auricular therapy is a gentle holistic treatment that has a clearing and soothing effect on the upper respiratory system via the links between the ears, eyes, nose and throat. This treatment also helps to clear the mind in preparation for deeper relaxation, e.g. meditation.

Special care

Care should be taken to encourage the right type of breathing for the right type of activity. Performing incorrect breathing contributes to conditions such as muscle cramps, headaches, depression, anxiety, tiredness and chest pains etc. as the exchange of gases is inadequate to meet the demands of the body.

Angel advice

Good breathing relies on good posture, which in turn affects good circulation. Bad habits such as crossing the legs should be avoided to prevent circulatory and postural problems.

- Lateral costal breathing constitutes normal breathing whereby the lungs take in enough oxygen to accommodate everyday activities.
- Apical breathing is shallow and rapid and is used by the body when maximum amounts of oxygen are needed to perform a strenuous activity. Breathlessness and fatigue occur when energy requirements exceed oxygen intake.
- Diaphragmatic breathing is deep and long, filling up the whole of both lungs with air and with it maximum amounts of oxygen. To perform this type of breathing, posture must be good and the body must be relaxed so as not to restrict air intake. This type of breathing should be encouraged during a reflexology treatment and can be accompanied with pressure to the solar plexus reflex on the breath in and a release of pressure on the breath out.

Case study

It makes sense to work the reflexes of the respiratory system after those of the skeletal/muscular systems. The head will have been worked generally when working the bones of the skull and face. Breathing and circulation will be improved which in turn will aid the rest of the body helping to bring about an increased state of overall balance.

Case study *(continued)*

Many clients suffer with respiratory problems in the form of allergies, congestion, stress etc. which in turn affects breathing. As a result, breathing is often increased, shallow and even laboured.

Working the respiratory system with pressure techniques can help to soothe irritation and unblock congestion with clients often experiencing the need to blow their noses, cough or even sneeze as a result. Their eyes may become watery as the system attempts to wash away irritation and congestion. They may need to yawn as the body becomes free to take in more oxygen. There can also be a psychological and spiritual cleansing taking place when working over this system, which may result in some form of release e.g. tearfulness, laughter etc. This system is associated with both the throat and the heart chakras, which are associated with communication and love, and as a result clients often feel the need to talk about their emotions.

As you learn to live reflexology, you may begin to feel a greater interconnection with your client during this stage of the treatment. Some practitioners may start to experience the physical, psychological and even spiritual feelings with their clients. You may experience the need to cough as you clear the communication channels of the throat, experience extreme emotions as you ease the tension in the chest or even feel the intervention of another force guiding you through the treatment. Try not to be alarmed – it is a natural part of the treatment and although it may take a little getting used to, it is evidence of the treatment working on many levels.

Task

Using the treatment card as a guide work over the reflexes on the feet, hands or ears. Mark down on the card when an area comes up. It may be that the client is alerted to the reflex by experiencing a tingling sensation, a slight pain or general discomfort in the form of tenderness etc. In addition, you may feel a tightness, puffiness, grittiness etc. in the corresponding area. Note this down by placing a mark in the corresponding box. You may want to tick or cross the box or even shade it in. By shading it in, you can shade part or the entire box to reflect what was felt. Make additional comments as you see fit. Remember to start with a consultation (new or updated). Continue with relaxation movements and treatment of the previous systems. Finish with relaxation movements, breathing exercises, feedback and relevant aftercare advice.

Knowledge review

1 Name the structures that make up the upper respiratory tract.

2 Name the structures that make up the lower respiratory tract.

3 What are sinuses?

4 Name the tube that links the nasal cavity with the ears.

5 What is the function of the adenoids and tonsils?

6 Which part of the respiratory tract contains the vocal cords?

7 Name the three types of breathing.

8 Where are the reflex points for the sinuses located on the feet?

9 In which zones are the lungs located on the hands?

10 What is the function of point zero of the ears?

Reflexes of the digestive system

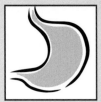

16

The digestive system begins at the mouth and ends at the large intestine and it is collectively known as the alimentary canal. The alimentary canal consists of the following structures:

- Mouth – comprising the hard and soft palate, lips, muscles, teeth, salivary glands and tongue. The mouth provides the starting point for the ingestion of food and fluid.

- Pharynx – linking the respiratory and digestive systems, the pharynx provides a passageway for the ingested food and fluid from the mouth into the oesophagus as it is swallowed.

- Oesophagus – a long muscular tube (approx 25 cms in length) extending from the pharynx to the stomach. It lies behind the trachea and in front of the spine. Its muscular layers contract to move the ingested food down in a peristaltic action through a ring of muscle known as the **cardiac sphincter** and into the stomach.

- Stomach – a j-shaped sac which lies under the diaphragm on the left side of the body where the next stage of the digestive process takes place. It contains folds or rugae that allow it to stretch out when full and contract when empty. At the end of the stomach there is a ring of muscle called the **pyloric sphincter** which controls the entry of digested food into the small intestine.

- Small intestine – a long coiled tube (approx 6 metres in length) which fills the bulk of the abdominal cavity. It is made up of three sections: the **duodenum,** the **jejunum** and the **ileum**. Absorption of nutrients from the digested food takes place within the small intestine.

- Large intestine – known also as the bowel, it is divided into five sections: the **caecum**, the **colon**, the **rectum**, the **anal canal** and the **anus**. The large intestine is responsible for moving the waste products of digestion through the system for elimination out of the body.

In addition to the alimentary canal, the digestive system also relies on three accessory organs:

- Liver – the largest internal organ of the body, lying below the diaphragm in the upper right section of the abdominal cavity. The liver is one of the most important links between body systems and has many functions, some of which are directly associated with the digestive system. Functions include filtering, detoxification and deamination of blood, storage of nutrients e.g. some vitamins, glycogen and iron, production of bile to aid digestion and the production of heat to maintain body temperature.

- Gall bladder – a pear-shaped sac located just above the duodenum and under the liver. It is connected to both the duodenum (the first section of the small intestine) and the liver by ducts. It receives bile from the liver which it stores until needed by the duodenum to aid in the process of digestion and absorption.

- Pancreas – a long thin organ lying across the abdominal cavity on the left side of the body. It has an endocrine function producing hormones associated with blood sugar levels and an exocrine function producing juices associated with digestion. These digestive juices pass from the pancreas into the duodenum via a duct.

Together the alimentary canal and the accessory organs perform many functions which in turn have an effect on the well-being of the whole of the body including: **ingestion**, **digestion**, **absorption** and **elimination**.

- Ingestion of food and fluid takes place in the mouth where it is checked for temperature by the sensitive skin of the lips, held within the mouth by the facial muscles, tasted by the papillae (taste buds) of the tongue, broken down by the teeth and the action of the jaw, bound together with saliva and formed into a bolus before being passed to the pharynx where swallowing takes place.

- Peristaltic action sends the bolus down the oesophagus, passing through the cardiac sphincter and into the stomach.

- Digestion also begins in the mouth and carries on in the stomach. In the mouth mastication (chewing) takes place which breaks down the food into a bolus. Chemical digestion takes place through the action of saliva in the mouth and digestive juices in the stomach breaking the food down further to form a semi-liquid known as chyme. This passes from the stomach through the pyloric sphincter and into the small intestine.

- Vital nutrients from the chyme are passed from the stomach and small intestine into the circulatory system for transportation around the body. Small amounts of water, alcohol and some drugs are absorbed directly into the bloodstream from the stomach and the rest of the nutrients are absorbed from the three sections of the small intestine. This process is aided by the secretion of bile

Tip

A bolus is a rounded mass of chewed food ready to be swallowed.

Fascinating Fact

The cardiac sphincter is a weak muscle allowing regurgitation of food from the stomach if necessary.

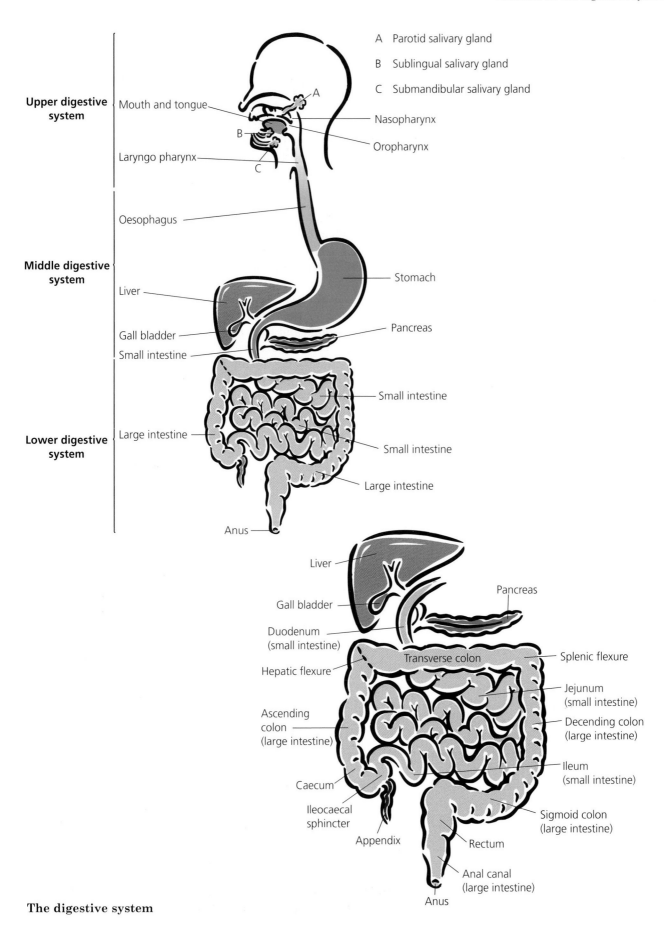

A   Parotid salivary gland

B   Sublingual salivary gland

C   Submandibular salivary gland

Upper digestive system

Mouth and tongue

Nasopharynx

Oropharynx

Laryngo pharynx

Oesophagus

Middle digestive system

Liver

Stomach

Gall bladder

Pancreas

Small intestine

Small intestine

Lower digestive system

Large intestine

Small intestine

Large intestine

Anus

Liver

Gall bladder

Pancreas

Duodenum (small intestine)

Transverse colon

Splenic flexure

Hepatic flexure

Jejunum (small intestine)

Ascending colon (large intestine)

Decending colon (large intestine)

Ileum (small intestine)

Caecum

Ileocaecal sphincter

Sigmoid colon (large intestine)

Appendix

Rectum

Anal canal (large intestine)

Anus

The digestive system

from the gall bladder and pancreatic juices from the pancreas.

- As the chyme reaches the latter stages of the small intestine any remaining matter forms into faeces. Peristaltic action forces the faeces along the rectangular colon from the ileocaecal sphincter linking the small and large intestines into the caecum, ascending, transverse, descending and sigmoid colon, through the rectum and into the anal canal for elimination out of the body via the anus. Any remaining water is absorbed along the way.

The healthy functioning of the digestive system contributes to the health of the whole body. Vital nutrients in the form of food and fluid are a necessary part of the survival of every cell, tissue, gland, organ and system in order to sustain life. These vital functions are often taken for granted as we expect our body to perform to optimum levels without providing a suitable environment in which to do so. The digestive system needs time to perform its functions and likes to do so in an environment of calm. All too often the body experiences a situation of overload as we try to combine functions – e.g. eating on the run – as a reaction to the stresses and strains of everyday life, leading to a stressed and strained system.

System sorter

DIGESTIVE SYSTEM

Nervous system

The nervous system picks up on the body's need for nutrients and initiates the feelings associated with hunger. The nervous system also picks up on the urge to release faeces from the large intestine. Failure to take note of these signs puts strain on the system.

Circulatory system

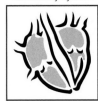

Nutrients are transported around the body within the blood for use by individual cells. Stimulating blood flow increases the efficiency of this process and ensures the efficiency of cellular function.

Integumentary system

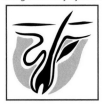

The skin produces vitamin D in response to sunlight. Vitamin D in turn aids in the absorption of calcium in the small intestine. Calcium is needed to maintain healthy bones.

Skeletal/muscular systems

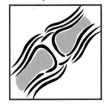

The jaw (maxillae and mandible) bones contain the teeth which contribute to the ingestion of food through mastication (chewing). The bones and muscles of the chest, back and pelvis together with the muscles of the abdomen help to protect the digestive system and its accessory organs.

Immune system

The adenoids, tonsils and appendix are all made from lymphatic tissue and aid the immune functions of the digestive system by filtering harmful substances. The adenoids and tonsils are located at the start of the alimentary canal within the throat and the appendix is located between the small and large intestines.

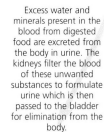

Oxygen from the lungs activates the glycogen from the digestive system to produce energy in the cells. Oxygen may be classified as a vital nutrient along with food and water.

Respiratory system

Excess water and minerals present in the blood from digested food are excreted from the body in urine. The kidneys filter the blood of these unwanted substances to formulate urine which is then passed to the bladder for elimination from the body.

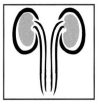

Genito-urinary system

The hormone adrenalin, produced in the adrenal glands in response to stressful situations, has the effect of temporarily shutting down the digestive system, diverting the blood to the muscles in order to activate the 'fight or flight' effect.

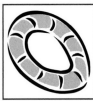

Endocrine system

Lymphatic capillaries and lacteals absorb fats from the small intestine before passing them on to the blood for distribution around the body.

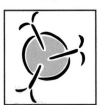

Lymphatic system

Mucus is produced along the linings of the alimentary canal by goblet cells in the epithelial tissue. This mucus helps the flow of nutrients and waste through the system.

Cells

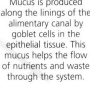

Consultation considerations

In order to ascertain the levels of stress the digestive system and its associated organs are under, it is useful to consider the following during the consultation process.

Oral

Many people suffer with a variety of symptoms relating to disharmony within the digestive system but find it very difficult to discuss. Care should be taken to ensure that the client understands what you are talking about by asking questions using commonly used words rather than technical terms that they may not be aware of. This avoids misunderstanding and embarrassment and leads to a greater awareness on the part of the practitioner and client. Be specific in your questions, giving ample opportunity for the discussion of symptoms explaining that this information will help in making the treatment more effective e.g. a person with constipation will benefit from a more stimulating treatment of the system than a person with looser bowel movements.

Useful exploratory questions can be asked with reference to appetite, digestion and elimination e.g.

- Enjoyment of eating?
- Regularity of meals?
- Symptoms of disturbed digestion e.g. flatulence, stomach cramps, bloated feeling, headaches, heartburn etc?
- Frequency of bowel movements?

Visual

Observing the overall build of a person i.e. under, over or average weight will give an insight into the activity of the digestive system as well as alerting the practitioner to the possibilities of associated problems e.g. strain on other systems associated with obesity and extreme underweight. The possibility of the presence of eating disorders may be highlighted at first sight and be mirrored in the results of the observation of the feet, hands or ears during the relaxation massage. The digestive system takes up a large section of the body and as such can be identified on the parts (especially the feet) well. Careful observation helps to determine further the actions of the system e.g. a dull, mottled pallor may be indicative of a congested system, a yellow tinge to the skin may indicate liver malfunction etc.

Aural

The digestive system is very responsive to changing emotions. It is therefore useful to try to pick up on the emotions behind the words a person is saying. Listening to the words as well as physically hearing them helps to determine the underlying emotions, which may then be linked back to the physical symptoms of the system e.g. the digestive system starts to shut down during extreme stress to allow the blood to be diverted to the muscles. As a result digestion is interrupted and disturbed. Nervousness, fear, anger etc. may be the stressors that activate this process and can be picked up in the way in which a client describes their symptoms, alerting the practitioner to the possible links. It may be that you also hear the sounds of a rumbling tummy etc.

Olfactory

Spicy foods, alcohol, coffee etc. may be detected in the smell of the breath. This may also provide a means of determining possible disharmony in the digestive system. In the case of foul-smelling breath, attention should be paid to the condition of the alimentary canal in its entirety during consultation and treatment to help to determine the possible causes, help to create balance within the system and encourage greater levels of awareness with aftercare advice.

Perceptive

Matching physical symptoms with emotions is an intuitive process that develops with experience. As well as providing an insight into the physical well-being of the body, the actions of the digestive system also provide a window into the psychological aspects of a person, e.g. constipation is a process of retention on a physical level that may be caused or be a contributory factor in the holding on of emotions. Conversely, regular bouts of diarrhoea may be associated with physical and psychological stress as a person experiences a need to let go of emotions. It will be necessary to call upon the skills of perception to begin to truly understand the possible causes and contributory factors relating to the well-being of the body as a whole rather than just that of the individual systems.

Tactile

The feel of the feet, hands and ears should reflect the workings of the system and the effects on the body e.g. obesity may be reflected in a puffy feeling where as extreme underweight may be reflected in a tight, empty feeling to the parts. Care should be taken to adapt the depth of pressure for both the client and the practitioner i.e.

- Suitable pressure to avoid undue discomfort for the client.
- Suitable pressure to allow detection of problem areas for the practitioner.

Contraindication considerations

Care should be taken to ensure that the information gained from the consultation is used for the adaptation of the treatment. There are no specific contraindications associated with the treatment of the digestive system with reflexology. However, activity within the system, i.e. just after eating, and severe symptoms of general or specific disharmony would need the application of well thought through adaptation of pressure to ensure an effective treatment. If in any doubt it is best to avoid the area until medical advice has been sought or until activity is lessened.

Reflexes

Applying pressure movements to the parts that make up the digestive system and accessory organs needs to be carried out with care and consideration. As with all systems, the digestive system may be treated generally or specifically and your course of study will direct you whilst experience will help you to develop a course of action suited to you and your clients.

The position of the reflexes

The digestive system takes up a large section of the body and can be seen to take up a large section of the parts suitable for reflexology treatment. The digestive system is located within each of the longitudinal and transverse zones and as such many practitioners will work generally over the feet, hands and ears. A more specific treatment of the system may also be considered working the upper, middle and lower sections in turn e.g. first on one foot then on the other.

- Mouth and throat – see respiratory system.
- Oesophagus – from the base of the big toe/thumb to the diaphragm line and the lower concha of the ear.
- Stomach – from diaphragm to waistline in zone 1 of the right foot and zones 1 to 4 of the left foot/hand and the heart of the concha at the base of the helix of the ear.
- Liver and gall bladder – from diaphragm to waistline in zones 3 to 5 of the right foot/hand and the upper concha of the ear.
- Pancreas – below stomach in zone 1 of the right foot/hand and zones 1 to 4 of the left foot/hand and the upper concha of the ear.
- Small intestine – from waist to pelvic line in zones 1 to 4 of both feet/hands and the upper concha of the ear.
- Large intestine – from waist to pelvic line in zones 1 to 5 of both feet/hands and the upper concha of the ear.
- Rectum and anus – in zone 1 on the left foot/hand at the medial edge of the pelvic line and the antihelix of the ear.

Digestive system – order of work

Tip

For treatment of the specific reflexes follow the corresponding numbers on the diagram.

Suggested order of work – feet

The reflexes for the first part of the digestive system, i.e. the mouth and throat, are worked during treatment to the respiratory system and do not necessarily need to be worked again.

1. *Oesophagus* – place the thumb pad on the base of the big toe (plantar aspect) facing downwards. Work down from this point to the diaphragm line. Repeat twice more.

The upper abdomen

Zones 1 to 5 diaphragm line to waistline.

- Place thumb pad on the diaphragm line at zone 1 medial arch.
- Work across the foot from zones 1 to 5 and slide back.
- Change hands and repeat working from zone 5 to 1.
- Work until the whole area has been covered in slightly overlapping rows.

This will ensure coverage of the following reflexes:

2. *Stomach*

   - Left foot zone 1 to 4
   - Right foot zone 1
   - Diaphragm line to waistline.

3. *Pancreas*

   - Left foot zone 1 to 4
   - Right foot zone 1
   - Below stomach.

4. *Duodenum* (first part of the small intestine)

   - Left foot zone 1
   - Right foot zone 1
   - Below pancreas.

5. *Spleen*

   - Left foot zone 4 to 5
   - Below diaphragm line.

6. *Liver*

   - Right foot zone 3 to 5
   - Below diaphragm line.

7. *Gall bladder*

   - Right foot zone 3 to 4
   - Base of liver reflex.

Tip

The spleen contributes to the immune functions of the body and is not a part of the digestive system. However, because of its location in the body it will be worked when treating this area.

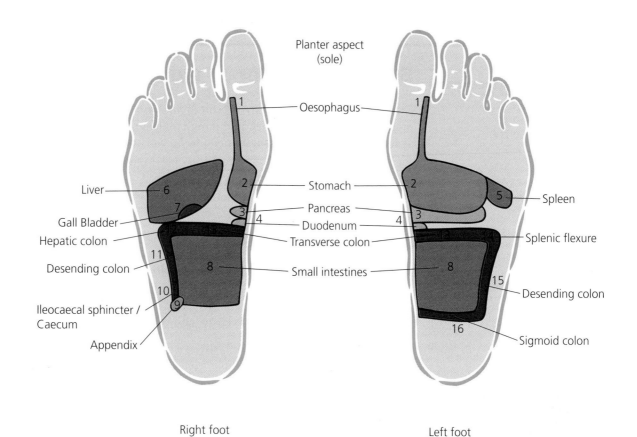

Planter aspect
(sole)

1 — Oesophagus

Liver — 6
Gall Bladder — 7
Hepatic colon —
Desending colon —
11
10
Ileocaecal sphincter /
Caecum
Appendix —
9
8

2 — Stomach
3 — Pancreas
4 — Duodenum
— Transverse colon
— Small intestines

1
2
5 — Spleen
3
4
— Splenic flexure
8
15 — Desending colon
16 — Sigmoid colon

Right foot

Left foot

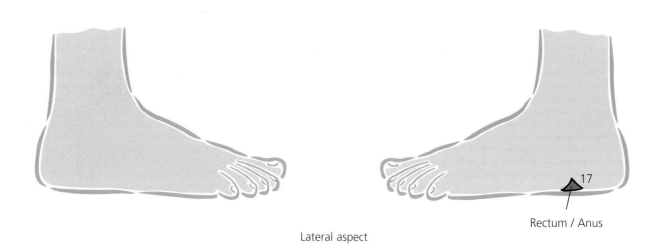

17
Rectum / Anus

Lateral aspect

The lower abdomen

Zones 1 to 5 waistline to pelvic line.

8. *Small intestine*

- Place thumb at medial arch at waistline
- Work across the foot from zone 1 to 5 and slide back.
- Change hands and repeat working from zone 5 to 1.
- Work until the whole area has been covered in slightly overlapping rows.

The large intestine

Start on the right foot.

9. *Appendix*

- Place thumb pad on the pelvic line facing towards the toes between zones 4 and 5. Pivot on the point.

10. *Ileocaecal sphincter / caecum*

- Move up with one small movement. Pivot on the point.

11. *Ascending colon*

- Work up towards the toes to a point just above the waistline.

12. *Hepatic flexure*

- Pivot on the point.

13. *Transverse colon*

- Turn thumb and work along waistline to zone 1.
- At the medial edge change to the left foot and work across from zone 1 to 4.

14. *Splenic flexure*

- Pivot on the point.

15. *Descending colon*

- Turn thumb to point towards the heel and work down to the pelvic line.

16. *Sigmoid colon*

- Turn thumb and work slightly above pelvic line to zone 1.

17. *Rectum / anus*

- Slide thumb out.

Tip

The appendix contributes to the immune functions of the body helping to protect the lower digestive system.

Remember

A flexure is a bend in the colon.

Suggested order of work – hands

The reflexes for the mouth and throat are worked during treatment of the respiratory system and as such do not need to be worked again.

1. *Oesophagus* – place thumb or index finger on the base of the thumb at the mid point facing downwards. Pivot on the point.

The upper abdomen

Zones 1 to 5 diaphragm line to waistline.

- Place thumb or index finger at the diaphragm line at zone 1 medial arch.
- Work across the hand from zone 1 to 5 and slide back.
- Change hands and repeat working from zone 5 to 1.
- Work until the whole area has been covered in slightly overlapping rows.

This will ensure coverage of the following reflexes:

2. *Stomach*
   - Left hand zone 1 to 4
   - Right hand zone 1
   - Diaphragm to waistline.

3. *Pancreas*
   - Left hand zone 1 to 4
   - Right hand zone 1
   - Below stomach.

4. *Duodenum*
   - Left hand zone 1
   - Right hand zone 1
   - Below pancreas.

5. *Spleen*
   - Left hand zone 4 to 5
   - Below the diaphragm line.

6. *Liver*
   - Right hand zone 3 to 5
   - Below the diaphragm line.

7. *Gall bladder*
   - Right hand zone 3 to 4
   - Base of liver reflex.

Remember

The spleen is worked at this stage because of its location.

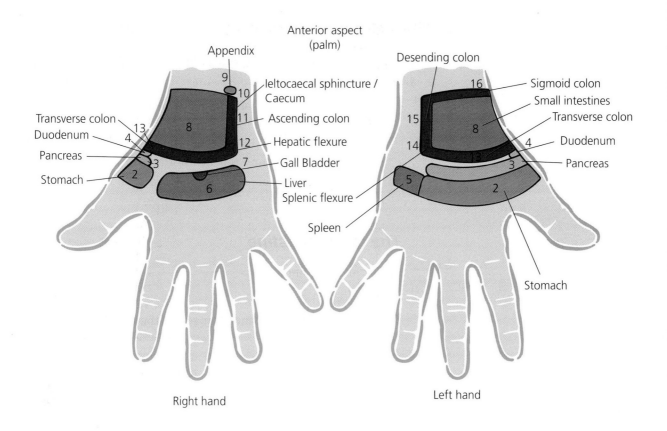

Anterior aspect
(palm)

Appendix

Desending colon

Ieltocaecal sphincture /
Caecum

Ascending colon

Hepatic flexure

Gall Bladder

Liver
Splenic flexure

Spleen

Transverse colon
Duodenum
Pancreas
Stomach

Sigmoid colon
Small intestines
Transverse colon
Duodenum
Pancreas

Stomach

Right hand

Left hand

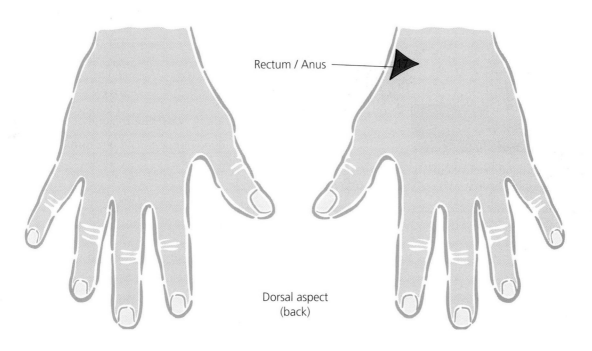

Rectum / Anus

Dorsal aspect
(back)

The lower abdomen

Zones 1 to 5 waistline to pelvic line

8. *Small intestine*

   - Place thumb or index finger at medial arch at waistline.
   - Work across the hand from zone 1 to 5 and slide back.
   - Change hands and repeat working from zone 5 to 1.
   - Work until whole area has been covered in slightly overlapping rows.

The large intestine

Start on right hand

9. *Appendix*

   - Place thumb or index finger on the pelvic line facing towards the fingers between zones 4 and 5. Pivot on the point.

10. *Illeocaecal sphincture/caecum*

    - Move up one small movement. Pivot on the point.

11. *Ascending colon*

    - Work up towards the fingers to a point just above waistline.

12. *Hepatic flexure*

    - Pivot on the point.

13. *Transverse colon*

    - Turn and work along waistline to zone 1.
    - At the medial edge change to the left hand and work across from zone 1 to 4.

14. *Splenic flexure*

    - Pivot on the point.

15. *Descending colon*

    - Turn towards the heel of the hand and work down to the pelvic line.

16. *Sigmoid colon*

    - Turn and work slightly above pelvic line to zone 1.

17. *Rectum/anus*

    - Slide out.

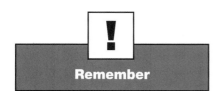

Remember

A flexure is a bend or curve in the colon.

Order of work – ears

Small pressure movements using the thumb to support the back of the ear and the index finger to work over the specific reflex points:

1. Oesophagus
2. Stomach
3. Pancreas
4. Liver
5. Gall bladder
6. Small intestine
7. Large intestine
8. Rectum/anus.

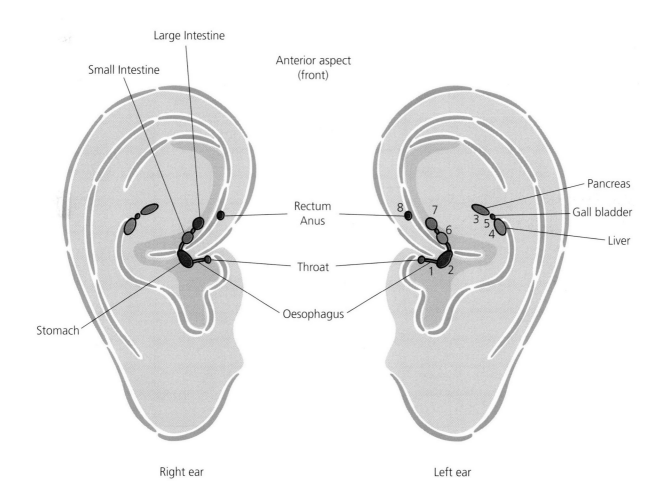

Right ear   Left ear

Treatment tracker

DIGESTIVE SYSTEM

Hands

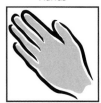

Feet

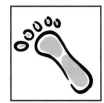

Ears

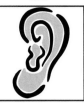

Visualisation

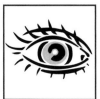

Affirmation

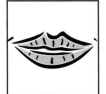

The digestive system takes up a large portion of the hands, starting in the thumb and ending in the lower section of the palm. Self-treatment is useful, especially for conditions such as constipation, where careful application of pressure techniques over the colon can help to aid elimination. It is important that movements follow the natural direction of the colon and that the area is not overstimulated.

The digestive system takes up a large portion of the feet, starting in the big toe and ending in the lower section of the sole. The use of pressure techniques over this area promotes deep relaxation and helps to open the energy channels between the body and mind. People often experience a freeing of emotions whilst this area is being treated.

The digestive system is located in the upper concha and helix region of the ears. It may be difficult to pinpoint the precise location of the specific reflexes, so general treatment of the whole of the ear concentrating on areas of tightness and discomfort will help to eliminate energy build-up which in turn will aid the elimination process of the body as a whole.

It is beneficial to have a working knowledge of the digestive system and its route through the body, and a poster is a useful addition to a treatment room in creating awareness ad helping in the visualisation process.
Try to visualise the energy from the universe entering the body and following the route of the digestive system. This energy must flow at an even pace throughout the system. If it is forced to slow down as it comes across blockages and congestion, try to imagine an extra force swirling around and easing them away. If it speeds up at any time, hold it back with your mind's eye until it eventually flows easy out of the body. This can be repeated until the energy is free-flowing peacefully at an even pace.

Digestive problems often accompany emotional problems and vice versa. The digestive system is automatically adversely affected by excessive stress because the physical shutting down process works in favour of other body systems, enabling them to deal with the stressor. As a result it is possible to lose sight of the natural flow of physical and psychological energy into and out of the body. Affirmations that positively assert the natural functions of the body are helpful, e.g. 'Time is the essence of free flow within the body; I have the body and I am willing and able to make the time.'

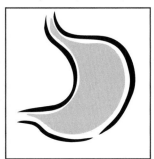

All of the chakras have an effect on the digestive system.
- The 7th chakra is associated with the thoughts and feelings surrounding the intake of food and fluid into the body.
- The 6th chakra is associated with the mouth, providing the entry point for food and fluid.
- The 5th and 4th chakras are associated with the pharynx and oesophagus and ingestion.
- The 3rd chakra is associated with the stomach, liver, gall bladder and pancreas and the associated functions of digestion and absorption.
- The 2nd and 1st chakras are associated with the small and large intestines with functions of elimination.

- The large intestine meridian starts from the index finger, ascends the arm, crosses the back of the shoulder and ends at the nose. It is stimulated between 5am–7am and calmed between 7pm–7pm.
- The stomach meridian starts under the eye, curves up to the temple and down the body to the top of the 2nd toe. It is stimulated between 7am–9am and calmed between 7pm–9pm.
- The gall bladder meridian starts at the outer corner of the eye, crosses the temple and descends to the shoulder, continuing down the outside of the body to the back of the 4th toe. It is stimulated between 11pm–1am and calmed between 11am–1pm. It is coupled with the liver meridian.
- The small intestine meridian starts at the little finger, ascends the arm, circles behind the shoulder and up to the cheek, outer corner of the eye and ends in the ear. It is stimulated between 1pm–3pm and calmed between 1am–3am and is coupled with the heart meridian.
- The liver meridian starts at the back of the big toe and ascends the leg and abdomen to the chest. It is stimulated between 1am–3am and calmed between 1pm–3pm. The liver and gall bladder meridians share the element wood.

The colour yellow is linked with the digestive system and is the colour of elimination. It has an effect on the liver and the intestines, helping to encourage purification through effective elimination. Skin problems respond well to effective elimination processes with the skin becoming blemish-free as a result. Yellow is also associated with the solar plexus and breath control which contributes to the elimination processes of the body.

The digestive system is located in all longitudinal and transverse zones. The upper part of the system extends down to the diaphragm line; the lower part of the system extends to the pelvic line. The accessory organs are located between the diaphragm and waistlines. Treatment of the digestive system through reflexology can be general, working the corresponding zones, or specific by following the digestive tract and its accessory organs to help balance and normalise its activity.

The note F is the predominant musical note associated with the digestive system and can be used to regulate its activities during reflexology treatment. However, because the alimentary tract emcompasses so much of the body, a variety of notes associated with each region will also have a therapeutic effect on the system and its parts. All types of classical music give the body access to a variety of notes in the format that suits the digestive system with louder, faster music creating a more stimulating effect than the quieter, slower music which will encourage a more calming and soothing effect.

Colour

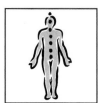

Chakras

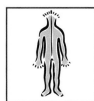

Zones

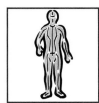

Meridians

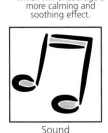

Sound

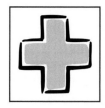

Common conditions

When treating the digestive system it is advisable to consider the effects it has on the other systems of the body and vice versa. A complete treatment is therefore advisable, paying attention to the reflexes directly and indirectly associated with the problem. Stress is a major factor in the well-being of the system and as such attention should be paid to the pituitary and adrenal glands, together with the solar plexus and respiratory system and the lymphatic and urinary system. The pituitary and adrenal glands are activated by stress, the solar plexus and respiratory system affect the amount of oxygen taken to the digestive system for the production of energy to perform its many functions and the lymphatic and urinary systems are contributory to the elimination processes. The list below gives common conditions and suggests direct and indirect reflexes.

An A–Z of common conditions associated with the digestive system

Activity

Work through each condition analysing the reasons for the direct and indirect reflexes. The list is not conclusive, so think of any more reflexes that may be associated and why.

- ACID REGURGITATION – a condition in which the contents of the stomach along with the hydrochloric acid from the gastric juices re-enter the oesophagus, causing it to become inflamed. *Direct reflex* = the cardiac sphincter. *Indirect reflexes* = stomach, oesophagus.
- ANOREXIA – avoidance of eating resulting in extreme deficiency and in severe cases death by starvation. It is a psychological disorder involving the fear of eating for any number of reasons. *Direct reflex* = the stomach. *Indirect reflexes* = small and large intestine, endocrine glands, kidneys.
- BOWEL CANCER – cancer affecting the large intestine. Can affect any part of the large intestine with growths that constrict the passageways. *Direct reflex* = the large intestine. *Indirect reflexes* = the rest of the digestive system and eventually the other body systems.
- BULIMIA – a disorder associated with over eating followed by self-inflicted vomiting and/or the use of laxatives. As with anorexia, bulimia is a psychological disorder and normal eating habits will only be resumed after the problem has been resolved. *Direct reflex* = the stomach. *Indirect reflexes* = small and large intestine, oesophagus, pharynx, mouth, teeth, endocrine glands, kidneys.
- CIRRHOSIS OF THE LIVER – hardening of the liver generally caused by the consumption of excessive amounts of alcohol. *Direct reflex* = the liver. *Indirect reflexes* = the whole of the digestive system, gall bladder and eventually other body systems.
- COELIAC DISEASE – an intolerance of gluten (a protein found in wheat). *Direct reflex* = the stomach. *Indirect reflexes* = small intestine, large intestine, thoracic spine.
- COLITIS – an inflammation of the large intestine resulting in diarrhoea combined with blood and mucus as damage to

the intestine lining occurs. *Direct reflex* = the large intestine. *Indirect reflexes* = small intestine, liver, gall bladder, pancreas, thoracic spine.

- CONSTIPATION – infrequent passing of waste from the anus resulting in dry, hard faeces as much of the water is absorbed making it increasingly difficult to pass. *Direct reflex* = the large intestine. *Indirect reflexes* = small intestine, stomach, liver, gall bladder, pancreas, thoracic spine.

- CROHN'S DISEASE – see ILEITIS.

- DIARRHOEA – abnormally frequent elimination of faeces during a peristaltic rush resulting in dehydration and weakness, as too much fluid and nutrients are lost from the body too quickly. *Direct reflex* = the large intestine. *Indirect reflexes* = small intestine, stomach, liver, gall bladder, pancreas, kidneys, endocrine glands.

- DIVERTICULITIS – inflammation of the large intestine resulting in abdominal pain and possible constipation. *Direct reflex* = the large intestine. *Indirect reflexes* = small intestine, stomach, liver, gall bladder, thoracic spine.

- FLATULENCE – air in the stomach or intestines that has been swallowed whilst eating or drinking. It may also be associated with certain foods, which produce a gas as digestion takes place. *Direct reflex* = stomach or intestines. *Indirect reflexes* = the rest of the digestive system.

- GALLSTONES – solid mass formation of particles of bile found within the gall bladder causing a possible obstruction preventing bile from passing into the duodenum. Extreme cases may lead to the complete removal of the gall bladder. *Direct reflex* = the gall bladder. *Indirect reflexes* = small intestine, liver, thyroid gland.

- GASTRITIS – irritation or inflammation of the stomach. Can be associated with something that has been eaten or drunk. *Direct reflex* = the stomach. *Indirect reflexes* = the rest of the digestive system.

- GASTROENTERITIS – inflammation of the stomach and intestines resulting in vomiting and diarrhoea. Dehydration and weakness can occur very quickly so care must be taken to replace lost fluid and nutrients. *Direct reflex* = the stomach. *Indirect reflexes* = small and large intestines, liver, gall bladder, pancreas, kidneys.

- HAEMORRHOIDS – a 'pile' or swollen veins in the anus causing pain and discomfort. Bleeding from these veins can result in anaemia due to the excessive loss of iron in the blood. May occur either outside or inside of the anal sphincter muscles. *Direct reflex* = the anus. *Indirect reflexes* = large intestine, thoracic and lumbar spine.

- HEPATITIS – inflammation of the liver. *Direct reflex* = the liver. *Indirect reflexes* = gall bladder, small and large intestines.

- HERNIA – a rupture (tear) whereby an organ penetrates its protective covering. A common site of a hernia is the large intestine in men. *Direct reflex* = the large intestine. *Indirect reflexes* = small intestine, stomach, thoracic spine.

- HIATUS HERNIA – a protrusion of part of the stomach through the opening in the diaphragm for the oesophagus (hiatus). *Direct reflex* = the stomach. *Indirect reflexes* = oesophagus, diaphragm, thoracic spine.

- INDIGESTION – pain associated with eating certain foods, which are more difficult to digest. It is also associated with over eating, hunger and other, often stress related disorders. *Direct reflex* = the stomach. *Indirect reflexes* = oesophagus, small and large intestines.

- ILEITIS – an inflammation of the latter section of the small intestine (ileum). Also known as Crohn's disease. *Direct reflex* = the small intestine. *Indirect reflexes* = stomach, large intestine, liver, gall bladder, pancreas, thoracic spine.

- IRRITABLE BOWEL SYNDROME – IBS – a condition commonly associated with high stress factors. Symptoms include alternate bouts of diarrhoea and constipation. *Direct reflex* = the small or large intestines. *Indirect reflexes* = stomach, pancreas, liver, gall bladder, thoracic spine.

- JAUNDICE – damage to liver cells resulting in a yellow discolouration of the skin and conjunctivae (the covering of the eyeball and lining of the eyelid). May be caused by infection, drugs or gallstones. *Direct reflex* = the liver. *Indirect reflexes* = gall bladder, small intestines, eyes.

- OESOPHAGITIS – inflammation of the oesophagus often associated with heartburn – a burning sensation in the chest. *Direct reflex* = the oesophagus. *Indirect reflexes* = stomach, small and large intestines, thoracic spine.

- OESOPHAGUS CANCER – malignant growths along the oesophagus. Most commonly found at the lower section of the oesophagus and occurs mainly in middle aged men. *Direct reflex* = the oesophagus. *Indirect reflexes* = stomach, small and large intestines, thoracic spine.

- PROCTITIS – inflammation of the lining of the rectum resulting in pain while passing faeces together with the urge to pass more. *Direct reflex* = the rectum. *Indirect reflexes* = large intestine, small intestine, thoracic spine coccyx.

- PROLAPSE – the displacement of a part of the body e.g. rectum. *Direct reflex* = the rectum. *Indirect reflexes* = large intestine, thoracic spine and coccyx.

- STOMACH CANCER – a malignant disease that is more common in men over the age of forty. *Direct reflex* = the stomach. *Indirect reflexes* = the rest of the digestive system and eventually other body systems.

- ULCERS – a break in the surface of any part of the body. Commonly associated with various parts of the digestive system where there is a break in the lining of the alimentary canal caused by the over production of acid in the gastric and intestinal juices. *Direct reflex* = the stomach. *Indirect reflexes* = oesophagus, small and large intestine, thoracic spine.

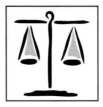

Holistic harmony

The digestive system and its associated organs provide the body with access to the nutrients vital for life from the intake of food and fluid. The organs of digestion rely on the system itself for their own survival as well as their links with other systems of the body. Additional factors contribute to the smooth running of the system and should be considered as part of the reflexology treatment and subsequent aftercare advice, encouraging a greater sense of awareness of the workings of the body together with an increased sense of responsibility.

Air

Oxygen breathed into the lungs is absorbed into the blood and, taken to the heart, where it is pumped to every cell of the body for the production of energy to facilitate cellular function. In addition to oxygen, every cell also requires nutrients from the digestive system. A lack of oxygen results in poor functioning at cellular level which in turn affects the functioning of the whole body, rapidly resulting in death. A lack of nutrients also results in a weakening of cellular function leading to a gradual degeneration of cells and eventual death.

Water

The intake of water is as important to the digestive system as it is to the body as a whole. Water is taken into the body via the digestive system and, absorbed into the blood as it passes through the stomach and intestines providing each cell with access to this vital commodity. However, the system itself relies on there being enough water present to avoid localised dehydration and resulting problems e.g. constipation results from the absorption of water from the faeces leading to a build up of dry, hard waste that is difficult and painful to pass out of the body. In addition, the build up of waste has a knock-on effect on other body systems, contributing to the sluggish appearance of skin when toxins held within the faeces are kept in the body longer than naturally intended.

Nutrition

The digestive system is responsible for breaking down the elements of ingested food so that digestion and absorption of nutrients can take place, providing the body with the means to sustain life. The nutrients essential for life include air, water and food. Food may be classified as **carbohydrates, proteins, fats, minerals, vitamins** and **fibre**.

- Carbohydrates – made up of three elements – carbon, hydrogen and oxygen – forming sugars that are broken down by the body to provide the fuel for energy production. Some sugars are water-soluble and as such are fast acting whilst others take longer to be absorbed and have a slow release action. Examples of fast acting carbohydrates include sugar, sweets and most fast food, providing the body with a quick fix. Examples of slow releasing carbohydrates include vegetables and fresh fruit, providing the body with a more sustained flow of energy.

- Proteins – made out of molecules called amino acids which contain nitrogen. Different combinations of amino acids make up the different kinds of proteins that are needed by the body for tissue growth and repair and the production of hormones, enzymes, antibodies and neurotransmitters. Proteins in the form of eggs, cheese, meat, fish, soya, lentils, peas and beans etc. are broken down, absorbed by the blood and taken to the liver. Here they are either used by the liver cells to form plasma proteins, transaminated (changed from one type to another), deaminated (those that are not required are broken down further and formed into the waste product urea) or sent out for use by the cells of the rest of the body. In the absence of other nutrients, the cells will use proteins as fuel.

- Fats – made of carbon, hydrogen and oxygen and form either saturated (hard) or unsaturated (soft) fat. Fats are absorbed into the lymphatic system via lacteals during the digestive process before entering the blood flow to provide the body with another source of energy which can be stored. Saturated fats are found in meat and dairy produce, are not essential and taken in excess, contribute to heart disease. Unsaturated fats in the form of monounsaturated e.g. olive oil and polyunsaturated e.g. nut and seed oils are a more useful source of fats.

- Minerals – essential for almost all cellular functions and contribute to the structure of bones and teeth. Some minerals are formed in the body whilst others (essential minerals) are supplied by the food we eat. Minerals needed by the body include relatively large amounts of calcium, magnesium, phosphorus, potassium and sodium. Other minerals are needed in much smaller amounts and are classed as trace minerals e.g. manganese, copper, chromium, zinc, iron and selenium. Surplus minerals are either not absorbed so lost from the body in faeces, or taken to the kidneys and lost through urine excretion.

- Vitamins – essential to life and form either water-soluble or fat-soluble nutrients. Recommended levels of these vitamins forms a complex equation that differs depending on the vitamin and its function and the specific needs of each person as they go through their life cycle. Water-soluble vitamins include vitamins C and B whilst vitamins A, D, E and K are all fat-soluble. The liver stores vitamins A and B12 and vitamins A, D, E and K are all stored in fat cells.

- Fibre – a tough fibrous carbohydrate that cannot be digested. Insoluble fibre, such as cellulose found in wheat bran, fruit and vegetables, adds bulk to the faeces allowing it to absorb water. This bulk stimulates peristaltic action in the large intestine, reducing the risk of constipation and infection.

Fascinating Fact

The body is made up of approximately 25 per cent protein. Think about the proteins (keratin and collagen) that make up the skin, hair and nails.

Ageing

Age affects the energy requirements of the body which tends to decline with age. As a result the body requires less food to sustain the decreasing levels of activity. The digestive system informs the body of the need for food via the brain, which alerts a person to eat with feelings of hunger. However, we often choose to ignore these signs and engage in erratic eating habits. We either over eat out of habit or boredom or under eat through lack of time and stress. There may even be additional strains that encourage us to either over or under eat that have a psychological and emotional root, as in the cases of eating disorders e.g. anorexia and bulimia.

Middle age is often accompanied by weight gain as the signs associated with decreasing energy levels are ignored. The weight gained during these years of life is more difficult to lose, as the digestive and absorption functions of the system also tend to decline with age. Care should be taken to ensure that throughout the stages of life, input of nutrients matches energy requirements to avoid excessive weight gain or indeed weight loss.

Rest

The digestive system requires a period of relative rest during the ingestion, digestion and absorption processes. Large amounts of blood are required to allow these processes to happen naturally and efficiently and as a result blood is diverted from other systems. If the body remains excessively active during or directly after eating, the blood is needed to sustain that activity, taking it away from the process of digestion. When this occurs, the body experiences symptoms of indigestion such as nausea, bloating, flatulence and stomach cramps. Periods of inactivity associated with the rest of the body are needed to allow for the increased activity within the digestive system until the processes are complete.

Periods of rest also provide the body with the time it needs to absorb, transport and store the various nutrients for availability and efficient use when needed. Subsequently, the elimination of waste occurs more efficiently after a period of rest.

Activity

Activity is made possible when the vital nutrients have been ingested, digested and absorbed and waste products eliminated. This is a continuous cycle as carbohydrates, fats, protein, minerals and vitamins are used for vital cellular functions to maintain a healthy body and waste products are produced as part of each process. The whole body replicates in a magnified manner the minute actions of each of the individual cells.

Ideally activity should match input of food in order to sustain a healthy, working body and avoid excessive weight gain or weight loss. As activity fluctuates so should food intake, bearing in mind the physical and psychological needs of the body. This activity requires each person to take responsibility for the well-being of

Angel advice

Gentle exercises performed well massage the internal organs and improve their functions.

their body and reflexology can help to create greater awareness and so positive action.

Awareness

The human body is made up of elements which form gases, liquids and solids. The elements oxygen, hydrogen, carbon and nitrogen form the major part of the body and are present in water, carbohydrates, proteins, fats and vitamins. The rest of the body (approximately 4 per cent of the total) is made up of minerals.

The cells of the body are continuously carrying out a variety of functions in order to sustain life, for which they rely on the food we eat and the fluid we drink. It is true to say that 'we are what we eat'. The quantity and quality of food and fluid therefore has a bearing on our well-being and needs serious consideration.

Being aware of how the body functions and what it needs to perform such functions empowers a person to take more control over their life. This awareness has the potential to lead a person to increased physical, psychological and spiritual well-being through loving and knowing. To love oneself is ultimately to know oneself and vice versa.

Children develop with an inbuilt awareness and sense of eating and drinking only when they need to until the boundaries of society are forced upon them. Our cultures' obsession with meal times and the traditions associated with what should be eaten when and with what imposes a set of guidelines that often go against the real needs of the body.

Special care

Caring for the digestive system results in the digestive system caring for the rest of the body. Care of this complex system should include:

- Regular meals to match energy levels.
- A balanced diet to maintain cellular functions.
- At least one litre of water per day to prevent dehydration.
- Fresh, unprocessed food for maximum nutritional value.
- Eating when hungry and not out of boredom avoids excess.
- Taking time out to eat aids digestion and absorption.

Consideration should be given to nutritional supplements during times of life when extra care is needed e.g. recovering from illness, pregnancy, ageing etc.

Fascinating Fact

The digestive system is often put under excessive strain caused by medication e.g. pain killers often result in constipation, anti-inflammatory drugs often upset the smooth working of the digestive system as a whole. The liver also has to work overtime helping to rid the body of the remains of the drugs.

Case study

Many clients seek reflexology treatment after experiencing problems associated with the digestive system and its accessory organs. As the functioning of this system is so reliant on peace and quiet, any form of stress has the potential to adversely affect it and so many people from all walks of life and of all ages find themselves experiencing increasing levels of stress in their lives. The digestive system is also at the root of a person's emotions and as such forms the seat of many psychological problems as people experience difficulties in holding on to or letting go of emotions. Thus the digestive system becomes the focus point for many physical and psychological disorders.

When following the suggested order of work, the digestive system benefits from the levels of relaxation already achieved from working on the skeletal/muscular and respiratory systems as well as the systemic systems. As a result, the subsequent pressure techniques are more effective and efficient. Many practitioners work the digestive system by treating each foot or hand in turn. The suggested method which may prove to be more effective is to work first the upper, then the middle and finally the lower parts of the digestive system in turn on both feet/hands simultaneously. This method tracks the pathway of the alimentary canal, stimulating the action in the parts in the order that they work naturally. In addition, working each part in the direction of its natural flow encourages better digestion, absorption and elimination and as a result congestion, e.g. constipation, can be freed and irritation, e.g. an irritable bowel, soothed. This is especially beneficial when any congestion or irritation is associated with the physical side effects of medication, change of water or diet etc. and/or the psychological effects of extreme emotions e.g. fear, anxiety or depression. Clients will often experience rumblings, accompanied by movement within the system and possible extremes of emotions as congestion is relieved. This is natural and should be viewed as a positive effect of the treatment rather than an embarrassing contra action.

It is also important to be aware that whilst it may be possible to feel and indeed relieve areas of congestion, at the same time it may be possible to pick up on the natural activity within the system according to the time of eating and the content of the meal, and adaptations of movements should be applied so as not to overstimulate. It is therefore important to respect the digestive system by not overworking it but also to be aware of the very real amounts of relief that treatment can bring at all levels.

Task

Using the treatment card as a guide, work over the reflexes on the feet, hands or ears. Mark down on the card when an area is tender, puffy etc. Note this down by placing a mark in the corresponding box. Make additional comments as necessary. Remember to start with a consultation (new or updated), and continue with relaxation movements and treatment of the previous systems. Finish with relaxation movements, breathing exercises, feedback and relevant aftercare advice.

Knowledge review

1   Name the parts that make up the alimentary canal.

2   What are the three accessory organs?

3   Name the four functions associated with the digestive system.

4   What is the name given to the muscular action that moves the food and waste through the system?

5   Name the parts that make up the large intestine.

6   What are the seven vital nutrients that are found in the food we eat?

7   How is digestion affected by stress?

8   Where is the stomach reflex located on the feet?

9   In which transverse zones are the small intestines located on the hands?

10   Where are the reflex points for the accessory organs found on the ears?

Reflexes of the genito-urinary system

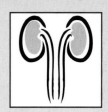

The genito-urinary system consists of the male and female **genitalia**, the **kidneys**, **bladder**, **ureter** tubes leading from the kidneys to the bladder and a **urethra** tube leading from the bladder to the outside of the body.

MALE

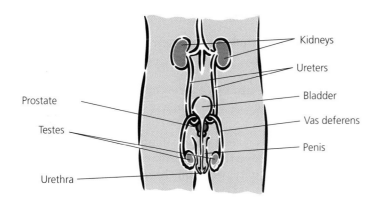

FEMALE

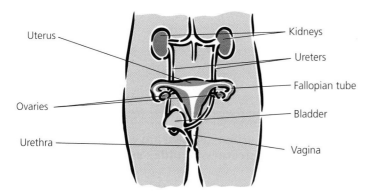

The male and female genito-urinary systems

Male genitalia

The male genitalia include the **testes**, the **vas deferens**, the **prostate gland** and the **penis**.

- Testes – develop in the abdomen of a male foetus and drop into a sac of skin and muscle located behind the penis, known as the scrotum, just before birth. After puberty the testes produce sperm which passes along a tightly coiled tube called the epididymis which extends to form the vas deferens.
- Vas deferens – peristaltic action forces the sperm along the vas deferens towards the penis. Each vas deferens passes by sac-like structures called **seminal vesicles** which secrete the fluid that mixes with the sperm to form **semen**. This fluid passes from the seminal vesicles to the vas deferens through ducts. Each vas deferens then passes through the prostate gland.
- Prostate gland – a chestnut-shaped structure which secretes a milky fluid contributing to the formation of semen. The prostate gland opens onto the urethra tube to create an exit out of the body through the penis.

Female genitalia

Remember

The female breasts develop in response to activity in the genitalia. They form above the pectoralis muscles and contain milk producing alveolar glands. These glands are activated into producing milk during pregnancy.

The female genitalia include the ovaries, the **fallopian tubes**, the **uterus** and the **vagina**.

- Ovaries – there are two ovaries on either side of the pelvic girdle about the size and shape of almonds, which store **ova** (eggs).
- Fallopian tubes – each approximately 10 cm in length opening just above the ovaries to create a passageway for released ovum to travel from the ovaries to the uterus.
- Uterus – or womb is the site for the development of an ovum which has been fertilised by a sperm or the release of the unfertilised ovum during menstruation. The uterus opens out into the vagina at the neck of the womb or cervix which together form the route for the birth of a baby.

Urinary system

The structures of the urinary system are common to both sexes and include the **kidneys**, **ureters**, **bladder** and **urethra**.

- Kidneys – there are two bean-shaped kidneys located either side of the spine at the waistline. The kidneys formulate urine which is passed out of the kidneys into the ureter tubes.

- Ureter tubes – two long, thin tubes extending from each kidney to the bladder. Peristaltic action forces urine along the ureter tubes.

- Bladder – a pear-shaped structure when empty, becoming oval in shape as it fills with urine. The bladder contains rugae which extend as the bladder fills. Nerve endings in the bladder wall detect an increase in size and activate an internal sphincter muscle which relaxes as the bladder contracts, allowing a passageway through to the urethra.

- Urethra tube – a single narrow muscular tube leading from the bladder to the outside of the body. It contains an external sphincter muscle closing off the exit to prevent release of urine. In a male the urethra is longer than in a female and has a dual function providing exit out of the penis for either urine or semen.

The functions of the genito-urinary system may be divided into two categories:

1. Functions of the genitalia which include the production of hormones and reproduction.

2. Functions of the urinary system which include filtration, reabsorption, production, excretion and regulation.

    - The testes and ovaries are also known as gonads or sex glands and are responsible for producing the male and female sex hormones.

    - The onset of puberty equips a male and female to reproduce a new human being with the production of sperm and the release of ova.

    - Large amounts of blood pass continuously through the kidneys to be filtered of unwanted substances. Many other vital substances are also filtered out of the blood during this process.

    - Reabsorption of these vital substances takes place prior to the production of urine as the kidneys regulate the amount of water and minerals needed by the body. The excess water, minerals and waste are then excreted from the body.

The dual functions of the genito-urinary system contribute to many vital functions of the body. The body gives out many signs that this system is working and will alert the body when stressed e.g. the feeling associated with needing to empty the bladder, sexual tension etc. All too often these signs are ignored and stress is allowed to build up, resulting in localised problems which in turn may develop into more general problems affecting other body systems.

System sorter

GENITO-URINARY SYSTEM

Nervous system

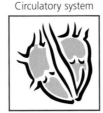

The nervous system alerts the body when the urine in the bladder reaches a certain level by activating the urge to pass urine. Reflex action in the external sphincter muscles prevents free flow until convenient.

Circulatory system

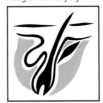

Excess water, minerals, hormones and waste products are carried by the blood to the kidneys for filtration and production of urine and eventual elimination from the body.

Integumentary system

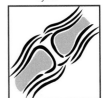

The skin loses water through sweating when body temperature rises. As a result, the kidneys reduce urine production to regulate fluid balance within the body.

Immune system

The avoidance and irregular passing of urine leads to a build up of toxins in the body putting extra strain on the immune system.

Skeletal/muscular systems

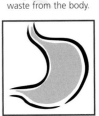

Bones and muscles offer protection to the organs of the genito-urinary system. Visceral muscular tissue is responsible for the passage of urine through the system, sperm from the testes to the urethra and ova from the ovaries to the uterus.

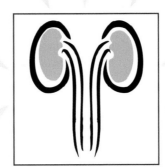

The action of breathing has the effect of massaging the internal organs of the genito-urinary system, helping to stimulate activity and maintain healthy functions.

Nutrients from the digestive system contribute to the formation of hormones in the testes and ovaries. Excess fluid from the digestive system forms urine aiding in the release of waste from the body.

Respiratory system

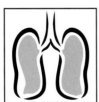

Transitional epithelial tissue which is contractible, forms the lining of the bladder, allowing it to expand when full of urine and deflate when empty.

The testes and ovaries are part of the genito-urinary system, as well as being endocrine glands secreting the male and female sex hormones responsible for the secondary sexual characteristics.

The lymphatic system is responsible for collecting excess tissue fluid, thus preventing oedema and fluid retention.

Digestive system

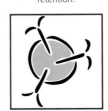

Cells

Endocrine system

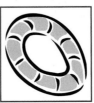

Lymphatic system

Consultation considerations

In order to determine the stress levels associated with the genito-urinary system, it is useful to consider the following during the consultation process.

Oral

Discussion of the functions of the genito-urinary system is usually met with an element of embarrassment on the side of both the client and the practitioner, and any questions asked should be treated with extreme care and sensitivity. With this in mind it is useful to ask a male client very open and general questions relating to their genitalia and reproduction, providing the opportunity for further discussion relating to potential problems – impotency, infertility etc. – without initiating it. Although female clients are often more accustomed to speaking openly about these parts of their body, any problems they may be experiencing can cause extreme distress.

Specific questions relating to this system may include:

Tip

If a client complains of passing blood in their urine it is important to refer them to their GP as there are likely be underlying problems that need medical attention.

- Any occurrences of common conditions e.g. cystitis, thrush?
- Fluid intake i.e. how much, how often and what?
- Pain or pressure when passing urine?
- Ask a female about regularity of periods and any associated problems.

Tip

Be aware of the fact that men over the age of forty may be prone to problems associated with the prostate gland.

More specific questions may follow with further treatments as a client becomes more accustomed to the process and more comfortable with the practitioner.

Remember

It is not necessary or indeed possible to find out everything about a client in one session. It takes time to build up a case history in much the same way as it does to build a relationship.

Visual

It is useful to take note of the general condition of the skin as this provides a window into the inner workings of the body. Changes in colour – yellowing of the part, differing texture – sweaty and wet or dry and grainy and lack of moisture – tight and wrinkly, may alert one to the possibility of problems related to the genito-urinary system which are often associated with varying levels of dehydration. Remember the majority of people do not consume adequate amounts of water.

Aural

The art of listening provides the key to many stress-related problems as underlying tensions and anxieties manifest themselves in physical problems. A client who says they do not have time to visit the loo, ignoring the signs their bladder gives out, is possibly saying a lot more than that they are busy. There may be an underlying problem at work i.e. fear of taking time out of a busy production process, or unrealistic demands being set resulting in a person's fear of showing any signs of weakness or inability to cope. Fear of pregnancy, childbirth or even having children can put excessive strain on a person, which may be picked up in the way in which they respond to related questions and sometimes in what is not being said. Listening to the silences is a useful skill that takes practice to perfect.

Olfactory

Odour is related to body functions as well as care of the body. Any odour detected provides an indication of these body functions as well as the way in which a person copes with them.

Perceptive

The consultation process provides a valuable insight into the well-being of a person. The way in which they respond to this process allows the practitioner to build a picture of each individual which develops as the treatments progress. It is important to be aware of the fact that each person is so much more than the sum of their parts and that lifestyle and life experiences play a huge part. Learning to understand the differences that make each person unique forms a vital part of the consultation process and an effective consultation will be one where the practitioner has tried to 'get into the shoes' of the client.

Tactile

Problems associated with the genito-urinary systems often stem from a diet lacking in adequate amounts of water as well as fluctuations in hormone production. The feel of the skin may be dry, tight and in some cases flaky and grainy. This is reflected in the feel of the feet, hands and ears and may be detected during the relaxation massage. The skin may start to desquamate (exfoliate) during the massage, resulting in a person feeling that they are discarding the old. This may relate physically but also emotionally as a person becomes more positive in their outlook with further treatment and aftercare advice.

Contraindication considerations

Care should be taken to consider the workings of this system and the times when stimulating it through reflexology may disturb the natural balance. It is true that reflexology is a natural process and as such there should be few contraindications. However, there are a few conditions to which caution should be paid including

- The early stages of pregnancy, especially if there is a history of miscarriage.
- During a heavy period.
- During treatment for infertility.

Reflexes

The reflexes of the genito-urinary system may be worked specifically to aid their individual functions e.g. production of urine in the kidneys and sperm in the testes etc., as well as those of the system of a whole e.g. excretion, production of semen etc.

The position of the reflexes

The position of the urinary organs is closely linked with those of the digestive system and may be difficult to locate without confusion. Experience coupled with a working knowledge of the anatomy and physiology of the systems and organs will help to make sense of the position of the individual reflexes.

- Ovaries/testes – outer edge of ankle and wrist and the helix of the ear.
- Fallopian tubes/vas deferens – across the top of the ankle/wrist and the helix of the ear.
- Uterus/prostate gland – inner edge of the ankle and wrist and helix of the ear.
- Kidneys – between zones 2 and 3 at waistline on the feet and hands and the upper concha of the ear.
- Ureter tubes – from the kidney to the bladder reflexes from waistline to just above pelvic line on the feet and hands and the upper concha of the ear.
- Bladder – medial edge of the feet/hands above pelvic line and the upper concha of the ear.

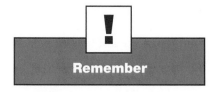

Remember

If during the consultation a condition throws any doubt as to the suitability of the treatment, it is always beneficial to gain medical advice with the client's permission.

Genito-urinary system – order of work

Suggested order of work – feet

- *Ovaries/testes* – place thumb or index finger on the central point between the protrusion of the outer ankle bone and the heel pad. Pivot on the point.
- *Fallopian tube/vas deferens* – using the thumb or index finger, work from the outer ankle to inner ankle across the crease line between the foot and leg. Repeat twice more.
- *Uterus/prostate gland* – place thumb or index finger on the central point between the protrusion of the inner ankle bone and the heel pad. Pivot on the point.
- *Kidneys* – place thumb pad on the waistline between zones 2 and 3 with the tip of the thumb facing towards the toes. Pivot on the point.
- *Ureter tubes* – swivel thumb around from the kidney reflex point so that the tip of the thumb is pointing towards the medial edge of the heel. Work down to the medial edge.
- *Bladder* – the bladder is visible as a slightly puffy area on the medial edge of the foot above pelvic line. Place pads of fingers or thumb over the centre of this area and work in a circular motion.

Tip

It makes sense to treat an organ in the direction of its natural function i.e. from the kidneys to the bladder and from the ovaries/testes to the uterus/prostate. This encourages greater free flow of urine, ova and sperm.

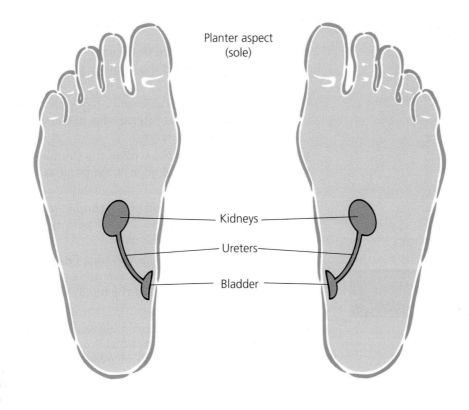

Planter aspect
(sole)

Kidneys

Ureters

Bladder

Right foot

Left foot

Joints

Fallopian tubes /
Vas deferens

Uterus / Prostate

Bladder

Medial aspect

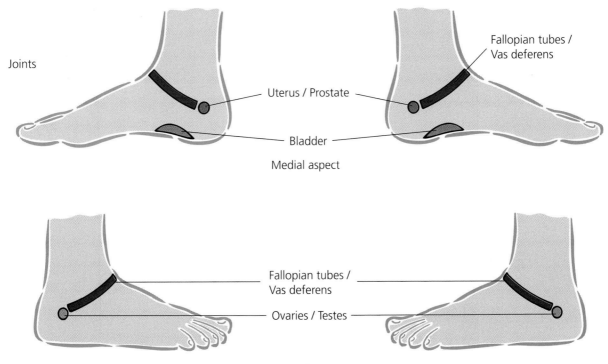

Fallopian tubes /
Vas deferens

Ovaries / Testes

Lateral aspect

Suggested order of work – hands

- *Ovaries/testes* – place the thumb or index finger on the dip in the lateral edge of the hand at the wrist. Pivot on the point.
- *Fallopian tubes/vas deferens* – using the thumb or index finger work from the lateral edge of the wrist to the medial edge. Repeat twice more.
- *Uterus/prostate gland* – place the thumb or index finger on the dip in the medial edge of the hand at the wrist. Pivot on the point.
- *Kidneys* – place the pad of the thumb or index finger on the waistline between zones 2 and 3 with tip facing towards the fingers. Pivot on the point.
- *Ureter tubes* – swivel thumb/index finger around from the kidney reflex point so that the tip is pointing towards the medial edge of the heel of the hand. Work down to the medial edge.
- *Bladder* – the bladder is visible as a slightly puffy area on the medial edge of the hand above the pelvic line. Place the pads of the fingers or thumb over the centre of this area and work in a circular motion.

!

Remember

To treat the organs in the direction of natural flow.

Anterior aspect
(palm)

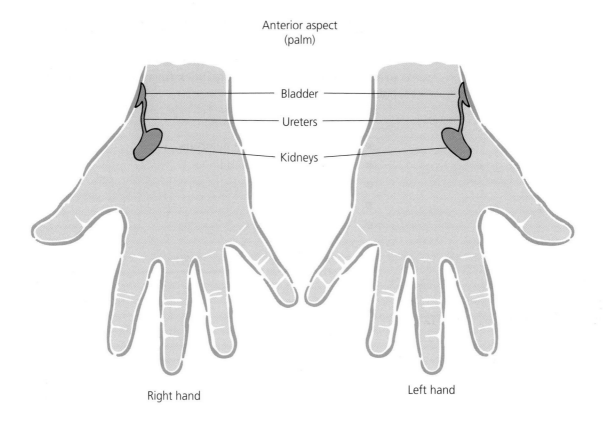

Bladder

Ureters

Kidneys

Right hand

Left hand

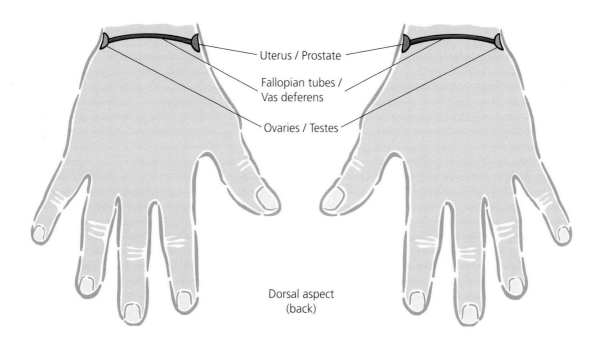

Uterus / Prostate

Fallopian tubes /
Vas deferens

Ovaries / Testes

Dorsal aspect
(back)

Suggested order of work – ears

With the thumb supporting the back of the ear apply small pressure movements using the index finger to the specific reflex points:

- Ovaries/testes
- Fallopian tubes/vas deferens
- Uterus/prostate gland
- Kidneys
- Ureter tubes
- Bladder.

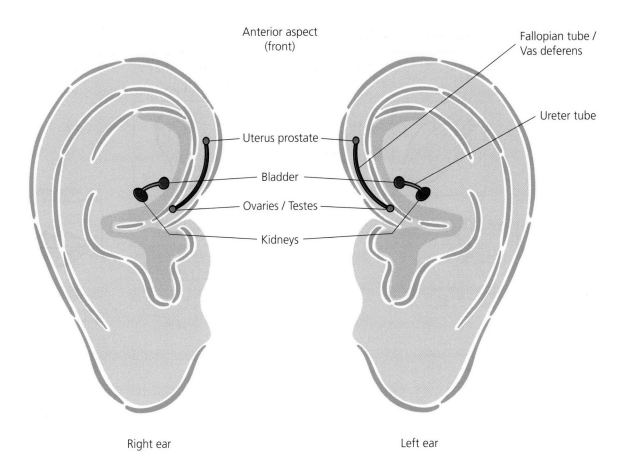

Anterior aspect
(front)

Fallopian tube /
Vas deferens

Ureter tube

Uterus prostate

Bladder

Ovaries / Testes

Kidneys

Right ear

Left ear

Treatment tracker

GENITO-URINARY SYSTEM

Hands

Feet

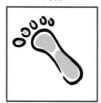

Ears

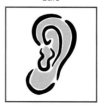

Visualisation

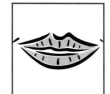

Affirmation

The genito-urinary system is located in the middle to lower sections of the hands. Observation of the hands with reference to the specific reflex points can help increase self-awareness. Dry skin over the urinary organs may indicate an imbalance in fluid levels. Puffiness over the genitalia will vary depending on life cycles e.g. menstruation.

The genito-urinary system is located in the middle to lower sections of the feet. The feet provide excellent access to the organs of this system, helping to regulate their activity. Complementary treatment can be offered for couples experiencing the early investigative processes associated with infertility, through this gently balancing and unobtrusive treatment.

The genito-urinary system is located in the upper concha of the ears. Self-treatment to the ears is a useful way of counteracting the potentially debilitating effects of stress. Treatment may be completed quickly, can be applied often and needs no special techniques. Self-treatment helps to encourage intuitive use of massage techniques resulting in greater self-awareness.

Visualisations help to create balance and free flow in a system that is associated with the physical flow of sperm, ova and urine. Visualise crystal clear, fresh water that is flowing naturally and gently. Imagine it creating a mirror image within the body, freeing any congestion associated with the genito-urinary organs. Now visualise bathing in the clear, bright light of the full moon as it gently cleanses and purifies the whole system. Be prepared to need to visit the loo after this visualisation as your levels of self-awareness increase!

Problems associated with the genito-urinary system are often related to the opposing forces of 'holding on' and 'letting go' at both a physical and psychological level. Holding on signifies a reluctance to release and letting go signifies a reluctance to retain. A balance between the two forces is the ultimate aim and affirmations can help to achieve this e.g. 'I am open to receive and free to release'.

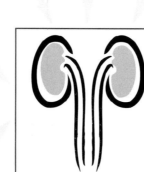

Red is associated with the genitals, blue is associated with the urinary system and orange activates the associated second chakra.

- The colour red has a stimulating effect on the genitals.
- The colour blue has a calming and neutralising effect on the system generally.
- The colour orange is associated with filtration and purification.

The second chakra has an affect on the genito-urinary system and is associated with the genitalia, kidneys, ureters, bladder and urethra. It is the energy centre associated with the perception of other people's emotions (clairsentience) and the point where sexual energy is sent out and received. The second chakra is also associated with the element water helping to cleanse and purify. The ritual of washing our hands before and after treatment reinforces this and can be seen as a means of cleansing away any remaining negativity to avoid transference from one client to the next.

The genito-urinary system is located within the waistline and pelvic line in zones 1–3. The kidneys lie in the upper part and the bladder in the lower part of the zone. It is sometimes difficult to be sure that you have located the kidneys when treating this system, as they are located within the centre of the body close to many of the digestive organs. It is useful to keep the image of the organ you are treating uppermost in your mind. This psychological focus will aid the physical aspects of the treatment, helping to create harmony and balance.

The bladder meridian starts at the inner corner of the eye, continues over the head, down the body and the back of the legs to the outer edge of the little toe. It is naturally stimulated between 3 p.m.–5 p.m. and naturally calmed between 3a.m. –5 a.m. The kidney meridian starts on the sole of the feet, ascends the back of the calf and the front of the thigh up the body to end at the chest. It is naturally stimulated between 5 p.m.–7 p.m. and naturally calmed between 5 a.m.–7 a.m. The yang bladder meridian is coupled with the yin kidney meridian, their associated element is water and their main function is to maintain normal fluid balance within the body.

The note C is associated with the genitals and the note D is linked with the urinary system. In addition, any type of flowing music is suitable for this combined system as is the sound of gently flowing water. The use of water in the treatment room in the form of a water feature can provide a natural way to encourage general free flow. The sound of water helps to stimulate physical and psychological elimination as well as calm and soothe the system generally.

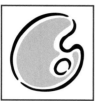

Colour

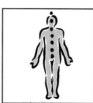

Chakras

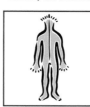

Zones

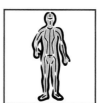

Meridians

Sound

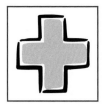

Common conditions

As body systems never work in isolation, it is always useful to carry out a full treatment to include all of the reflexes, paying particular attention to those *directly* associated with a problem as well as those *indirectly* involved. Treating the body in this way ensures harmony and helps to relieve the stresses associated with everyday living. When treating problems associated with the genito-urinary system the pituitary, adrenal glands, brain and associated spinal nerves and solar plexus reflexes will be affected due to their reactions to stress.

Tip

Common medical procedures associated with the genito-urinary system include:

- D&C – dilation and curettage. Involves the scraping of the walls of the uterus.
- Hysterectomy – removal of the uterus.

The list below gives common conditions and suggests direct and indirect reflexes.

An A–Z of common conditions associated with the genito-urinary system

Activity

Check the direct and indirect reflexes for six conditions of your choice. Do you agree with the direct and indirect reflex points? Can you think of any more?

- AMENORRHOEA – absence of menstruation caused by an imbalance of hormones. *Direct reflex* = the ovaries. *Indirect reflexes* = uterus, fallopian tubes, pineal gland.
- ANDROPAUSE – male menopause caused by decreasing male sex hormones often resulting in anxiety, depression and associated with the mid-life crisis scenario. *Direct reflex* = the testes. *Indirect reflexes* = prostate, vas deferens, pineal gland, liver, kidneys.
- CANCER – the development of malignant cells e.g. breast cancer, ovarian cancer, bladder cancer etc. *Direct reflex* = the affected area. *Indirect reflexes* = associated areas, thymus gland, spleen, liver, kidneys, lymphatic nodes and eventually the other systems.
- CERVICAL EROSION – changes in the lining of the neck of the womb accompanied by a slight discharge. *Direct reflex* = the uterus. *Indirect reflexes* = ovaries, fallopian tubes.
- CYSTITIS – inflammation of the bladder resulting in a frequent urge to pass urine with subsequently small quantities of urine being passed, often accompanied by

stinging and pain in the lower abdomen. A common complaint, which usually affects women more than men due to the difference in the size of the urethra. In women, the urethra is shorter and bacteria can enter the bladder more easily. *Direct reflex* = the urethra. *Indirect reflexes* = bladder, ureters, kidneys, lymphatic nodes, thymus gland.

- DYSMENORRHOEA – painful periods caused by hormone imbalance or may be associated with other disorders e.g. fibroids. *Direct reflex* = the ovaries. *Indirect reflexes* = uterus, fallopian tubes, pineal gland.

- ENDOMETRIOSIS – cells from the uterus form in the fallopian tubes or ovaries, causing pain especially during menstruation due to their response to hormone release. *Direct reflex* = the affected area. *Indirect reflexes* = associated areas, liver, hip.

- FIBROIDS – non cancerous growths which develop in the walls of the uterus. If large enough, can press on the bladder causing pain. *Direct reflex* = the uterus. *Indirect reflexes* = ovaries, fallopian tubes, bladder.

- IMPOTENCE – inability in a man to initiate or maintain an erection until ejaculation. The cause may be either physical and/or psychological. *Direct reflex* = the reproductive organs. *Indirect reflexes* = thyroid gland.

- INCONTINENCE – inability to control the external sphincter muscle of the urethra. May accompany urinary and prostate disorders and/or a weakening of the muscle due to excess pressure e.g. pregnancy and childbirth. *Direct reflex* = the urethra. *Indirect reflexes* = bladder, ureters, kidneys, prostate gland, uterus.

- INFERTILITY – inability of a woman to conceive or of a man to bring about conception. *Direct reflex* = the ovaries or testes. *Indirect reflexes* = uterus or prostate, fallopian tubes or vas deferens, pineal gland, thyroid gland.

- KIDNEY STONES – formed by an excess of salts in the blood. These salts crystallise in the urine and can cause an obstruction to the flow of urine resulting in extreme pain. Large stones may be surgically removed with small stones passing out of the body in urine. *Direct reflex* = the kidneys. *Indirect reflexes* = ureters, bladder, urethra, lymphatic nodes, thymus gland.

- MASTITIS – tender lumps present in the breasts of females associated with the lead up to menstruation. *Direct reflex* = the breasts. *Indirect reflexes* = ovaries, fallopian tubes, uterus, axillary nodes.

- MENOPAUSE – reduction in female sex hormones leading to the cessation of the menstrual cycle. Often accompanied by hot flushes, headaches, depression, mood swings etc. *Direct reflex* = the ovaries. *Indirect reflexes* = uterus, fallopian tubes, pineal gland, bones and joints, liver, kidneys.

- MENORRHAGIA – heavy periods lasting more than seven days, due generally to hormone imbalance but may accompany other disorders e.g. endometriosis, miscarriage etc. *Direct reflex* = the uterus. *Indirect reflexes* = ovaries, fallopian tubes, pineal gland, liver.

- MORNING SICKNESS – nausea and vomiting which sometimes occurs in early pregnancy. *Direct reflex* = the stomach. *Indirect reflexes* = ovaries, uterus, thyroid gland, oesophagus.

- NEPHRITIS – an inflammation of the glomerulus inside the kidneys. Nephritis can be either acute or chronic. In cases of acute nephritis the symptoms last for two to three weeks, often following an acute throat infection. Chronic nephritis may lead to kidney failure. *Direct reflex* = the kidneys. *Indirect reflexes* = ureter tubes, bladder, urethra, phayrnx.

- OVARIAN CYSTS/POLYPS – growths of tissue containing fluid on or around the ovaries. Can cause irregular periods. *Direct reflexes* = the ovaries. *Indirect reflexes* = uterus, fallopian tubes.

- PRE-MENSTRUAL TENSION (PMT) – physical and psychological tension leading up to menstruation caused by an imbalance in hormones. *Direct reflex* = the ovaries. *Indirect reflexes* = uterus, fallopian tubes, pineal gland.

- PROSTATITIS – inflammation of the prostate gland. *Direct reflex* = the prostate gland. *Indirect reflexes* = vas deferens, thymus gland, lymphatic nodes.

- PYELONEPHRITIS – inflammation of the kidneys due to an infection. There are two types – acute which may last a few days, and chronic which can last for many years and if left untreated cause kidney failure and death. *Direct reflex* = the kidneys. *Indirect reflexes* = ureter tubes, bladder, urethra.

- SEXUALLY TRANSMITTED DISEASES – a variety of diseases acquired through sexual contact. *Direct reflex* = the uterus or prostate. *Indirect reflexes* = vas deferens or fallopian tubes, ovaries or testes, thymus gland.

- THRUSH – an infection of the vagina. Symptoms include itchiness and discharge. *Direct reflex* = the uterus. *Indirect reflexes* = fallopian tubes, thymus gland, urethra, anus.

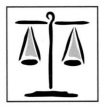

Holistic harmony

The genito-urinary system consists of two very closely linked systems which rely heavily on a balanced network between the other systems of the body to maintain their functions. As a team they share organs and as separate systems they contribute to the healthy development of the human race. Their needs are great and should not be ignored.

Air

As air temperature differs from season to season and country to country, the kidneys help to regulate the water and mineral balance within the body. When air temperature rises the amount of water lost by the body through sweat increases and as a result more minerals are also lost. The kidneys help to regulate the amount lost by reducing urine production. The body is naturally very adaptable but it can take up to ten days for it to acclimatise to a new environment where an extreme change in air temperature is experienced.

Water

The nervous and endocrine systems control the activity within the kidneys in response to changing fluid levels within the body. The brain picks up on any loss of water and alerts the endocrine system. In response, the pituitary gland secretes an **anti-diuretic hormone (ADH)**, to the kidneys. The kidneys in turn control the balance between the water going into the body and the water leaving the body. Water enters the body through the food we eat and the fluid we drink. Water leaves the body through expired air, sweat, urine and faeces as well as being present within tears, mucus and blood. When the balance is uneven either more or less urine is produced in the kidneys in order to rectify the situation. The brain also alerts the body to signs of dehydration by activating the sensations associated with thirst. However, the body can only give out the signal, each individual is then responsible for acting upon it! The body as a whole relies on water to maintain its many functions and a lack of adequate water results in localised problems which if not rectified develop into more serious problems. Surprisingly, research has now found that one of the last signs of dehydration is having a dry mouth!

Nutrition

Water is found in many of the foods we eat, providing an additional source which is often ignored or underestimated:

- Carbohydrates help the muscles store the water in which glycogen is bound.
- Fibre absorbs water making the passing of faeces easier.
- Fruit and vegetables contain large percentages of water as well as vital nutrients.

Other food sources have a detrimental effect on water balance including:

- Excessive salt encourages localised retention of water leading to oedema.
- Caffeine and alcohol act as diuretics encouraging the body to release more water.

A glass of water at the start and/or end of the reflexology treatment reinforces good practice and encourages a more positive result.

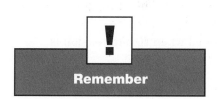

Males also experience a form of menopause which the medical profession have recently named **andropause**.

Always ask the client if they would like to visit the toilet before the start of the treatment to avoid the discomfort of a full bladder.

It is important never to give a person false hope in the treatment of their problem.

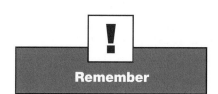

It is important to remember that reflexology cannot provide a cure for any condition, just a means to activate the body's own natural healing mechanisms.

Ageing

The genito-urinary system responds to the ageing process of the body, with certain functions being underdeveloped at birth. The reflex action associated with holding off the passing of urine develops in a young child. This situation may be reversed as the sphincter muscle weakens with age.

Reproductive functions are largely determined by age with puberty and menopause signalling the start and end of a person's reproductive years. The average age for puberty in boys is 13–16 and in girls 10–14. The average age for the onset of menopause in females is between the ages of 45–55.

Rest

Rest provides the body time to rebalance. Urine production is reduced during sleep, enabling the body to utilise the water over a period of time. However, rest will be disturbed if the body's need to consume or release water is too great!

In addition, hormonal secretions in the ovaries and testes result in changing energy levels which need to be rebalanced with periods of rest. Times of excessive internal function e.g. puberty, pregnancy, menstruation, menopause etc. require the body to indulge in more periods of rest.

Activity

Periods of activity stimulate all systems through increased blood flow. The massage associated with reflexology treatment is an activity that helps to stimulate in a controlled manner depending on length, depth and frequency of treatment. This controlled stimulation can help to balance stressed systems without placing any excess pressure on them. The genitalia and functions associated with reproduction can benefit greatly from this controlled stimulation, which helps with heavy and irregular periods, impotence and infertility.

Activity can also help to strengthen muscles that naturally weaken with age. This is of particular importance for the external sphincter muscle of the urethra and regular exercise can help to prevent the problems associated with incontinence.

Awareness

Children are naturally and intuitively aware of what their body needs and when, and if left to their own devices, with adequate facilities, will maintain their bodies in perfect working order. However, our culture forces us to exert control over when and where we perform certain bodily functions. Busy lives and lack of time add to the strain of performing such functions at necessary times and the body suffers as a result.

- A build up of toxins accompanies the build up of urine in the system when it is not regularly released.
- Relationships become strained when sexual tension is allowed to build up.

Recognising our own needs as well as being aware of the needs of others helps us to view the bigger picture that is life itself.

Special care

Efficient breathing, a balanced diet, good posture and positive thinking contribute to the well-being of all body systems including the genito-urinary system.

- Efficient breathing ensures adequate amounts of oxygen reach the cells needed to perform the necessary functions throughout life. Breathing also helps to massage the internal organs aiding peristaltic action.
- A balanced diet that is adapted to meet the physical and psychological needs of an individual ensures fluid levels are kept balanced and functions maintained.
- Good posture allows the internal organs to sit comfortably within the body without excess strain. Good posture during pregnancy is therefore very important.
- Positive thinking links body and mind, ensuring an overall balance helping at times of change e.g. puberty, pregnancy and menopause as well as having an effect on conception.

These considerations constitute a form of care that is in one sense special yet in another an absolute necessity.

!

Remember

The body is made up of a large percentage of water and as such, water is needed to maintain vital functions e.g. blood and lymph flow etc.

Case study

One of the increasingly common reasons for seeking reflexology treatment is for infertility, and the advice given to couples seeking medical treatment in the early stages is to relax and not to worry. This, however, is much easier said than done and many people (women in particular) will turn to complementary treatments as a means of doing something positive. The initial purpose of the reflexology treatment is relaxation and care should be taken to ensure that all the body systems are treated to begin to establish a level of balance. Weekly treatments to establish the activity associated with a woman's menstrual cycle e.g. length of cycle, associated pain, PMS, breast discomfort etc. is a suitable recommendation. As such, regular treatment can help to regulate the menstrual cycle as well as provide a means to ease congestion and stimulate function in the genito-urinary

▶

Case study (continued)

systems of both males and females. Regular treatment also encourages greater levels of self-awareness and many women start to experience a natural inkling of ovulation times as they become more aware of their bodies and associated cycles.

Treatment may also provide the opportunity for the exploration of inner feelings as both men and women come to terms with the possible psychological blocks they may be subconsciously exerting. Aftercare advice becomes a crucial part of the progressive treatment and there are many positive ways in which to help to counteract the negativity that a client may be experiencing at such a time e.g. the use of affirmations, visualisations as well as experimenting with colour and sound. I often encourage such clients to use these means to develop their nurturing skills on themselves and their partner as well as on any future children they may have. Self-love and that of those closest to us is often mislaid in times of stress, as many people seem to sink into themselves taking a very insular view of life, often finding it difficult to see the bigger picture. However, it is important to avoid any element of false hope as the reflexology treatment can in no way cure infertility. It is at best helping to create natural balance and harmony whilst encouraging the body to activate its own healing mechanisms. Reflexology can also be used to enhance the effects of infertility treatments but must be used with caution and in accordance with medical advice. Treatment may also provide a source of help with the feelings of despair, sadness, disappointment and failure that often accompany failed IVF treatment, miscarriage and impotence as well as infertility, helping to soothe the physical and psychological wounds. Care must be taken to avoid personal distress on the part of the practitioner as you become increasingly connected to your client and their situation. Be aware of your limits and work within them at all times.

Task

Using the treatment card as a guide, work over the reflexes on the feet, hands or ears. Mark down on the card when an area comes up i.e. is tender, puffy, grainy etc. Think about the reasons why. Remember to begin with a consultation (new or updated), continue with relaxation movements and treat the previous systems for practice. Finish with relaxation movements, breathing exercises, feedback and aftercare advice.

Knowledge review

1   Name the structures that make up the male and female genitalia.

2   Name the urinary organs.

3   What are the two functions of the genitalia?

4   Give three functions of the urinary system.

5   Give two contraindication considerations relating to the genito-urinary system.

6   How does the hormone ADH help to regulate fluid balance in the body?

7   What is the common age for the onset of puberty and menopause in females?

8   Where are the reflex points located on the feet for the male and female genitalia?

9   Where on the hands can the bladder reflex be found?

10   In which part of the ear are the urinary organs located?

Reflexes of the endocrine system

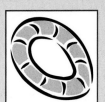

18

The endocrine system is closely linked to the nervous system. Together they act as communication centres of the body. The nervous system communicates its messages via electrical impulses and the endocrine system communicates with chemical messengers in the form of hormones. The nervous system is fast acting with immediate responses, e.g. reflex actions, whilst the endocrine

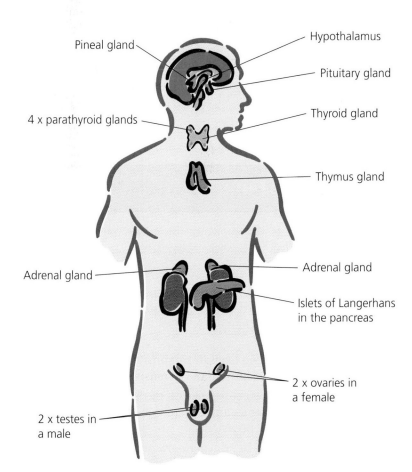

Pineal gland

Hypothalamus

Pituitary gland

4 x parathyroid glands

Thyroid gland

Thymus gland

Adrenal gland

Adrenal gland

Islets of Langerhans in the pancreas

2 x ovaries in a female

2 x testes in a male

The endocrine glands

system is more slow acting and responsible for gradual changes within the body e.g. growth.

The endocrine system consists of a set of ductless glands which are widely spaced around the body with each one being responsible for the production of hormones.

A hormone is a chemical substance formed from the components of the food we eat and are either protein-based or fat-based. Hormones have the ability to affect changes in other cells and are secreted directly into the bloodstream and transported to the various systems of the body. Target cells receive the hormones and allow the body to respond to the message and initiate the appropriate changes.

Endocrine glands and their hormones

Pituitary gland

Situated at the base of the brain behind the nose and consists of two lobes – the anterior (front) and posterior (back) lobes.

Anterior lobe – produces hormones that control other endocrine glands and other body systems:

- ACTH adrenocorticotrophic hormone – controls the cortex of the adrenal gland.
- TSH thyroid stimulating hormone (thyrotrophin) – controls the thyroid gland.

 Fascinating Fact

The pituitary gland is also known as the 'master gland' because of its controlling effect on the other glands.

- Gonadotrophins FSH (follicle stimulating hormone) and LH (luteinising hormone) – control the ovaries and testes.
- GH growth hormone (somatotrophin) – promotes growth of the skeletal and muscular systems.
- PRL prolactin – promotes growth of the ovaries, testes and mammary glands and stimulates lactation (milk production) in the breasts.
- MSH melanocyte stimulating hormone – promotes the production of melanin (colour pigment) in the skin.

Posterior lobe – produces two hormones that have an effect on the kidneys and the reproductive organs in females.

- ADH antidiuretic hormone (vasopressin) – decreases urine production by the kidneys to regulate fluid balance.
- OT oxytocin – stimulates the uterine and mammary gland contraction in preparation for childbirth and breastfeeding.

Pineal gland

Situated deep within the brain between the cerebral hemispheres. It is often referred to as the third eye because of its position. Responsible for the hormone melatonin, also known as 'the chemical expression of darkness' as it is produced at night in response to fading daylight.

- Melatonin – regulating the daily sleep/wake cycle, monthly menstrual cycle and body rhythms.

Thyroid gland

Situated just below the larynx and in front of the trachea in the neck. Consists of two lobes and is responsible for the secretion of three hormones in response to the production of TSH in the pituitary gland:

- Thyroxine and Triiodothyronine – regulate metabolism.
- Calcitonin – helps to maintain calcium and phosphorus levels by stimulating the storage of calcium and phosphorus in the bones and the release of excess in urine.

Parathyroid glands

Situated in two pairs on either side of the back of the lobes of the thyroid gland. Responsible for assisting the thyroid gland in the regulation of calcium and phosphorus levels with the production of parathormones:

- PTH parathormone – stimulates the reabsorption of calcium and phosphorus from the bones when levels in the body are low, and decreases the amount lost in urine.

Thymus gland

Situated behind the sternum in between the lungs. It is made of lymphatic tissue contributing to the immune functions of the body by producing a group of hormones called thymosins:

- Thymosin – stimulates the production of T-lymphocytes to protect the body against antigens (harmful substances).

Adrenal glands

Situated on top of each kidney. Each gland consists of an outer cortex and inner medulla:

Cortex – produces hormones known as steroids in response to the production of ACTH in the pituitary gland:

- Glucocorticoids including cortisol and cortisone – stimulating metabolism, development and inflammation.
- Mineralocorticoids including aldosterone – regulating mineral concentration in the body.
- Gonadocorticoids including androgens – stimulating sexual development.

Medulla – produces stress hormones in response to stimulation by the sympathetic nervous system to prepare the body for fight or flight:

- Adrenalin and noradrenalin – responsible for stimulating body systems needed for physical action e.g. muscular and respiratory, and shutting down those not needed e.g. digestive and urinary.

Islets of Langerhans

Situated in small clusters at irregular intervals within the pancreas. Responsible for the regulation of blood sugar levels with the production of two hormones:

- Insulin – reduces blood sugar levels by promoting the storage of excess sugar (glycogen) in the liver and muscles.
- Glucagon – increases blood sugar levels by promoting the release of sugar (glycogen) from the liver and muscles.

Ovaries

Situated within the female pelvic girdle on either side of the uterus (see genito-urinary system Chapter 17). Responsible for the secretion of female sex hormones:

- Oestrogen and progesterone – responsible for the development of secondary sexual characteristics e.g. menarche (start of menstruation), development of breasts, widening of hips and the growth of pubic and axillary hair.

Testes

Situated in the male scrotum which hangs externally from the body under the penis (see genito-urinary system Chapter 17). Responsible for the secretion of the male sex hormone:

- Testosterone – responsible for the development of secondary sexual characteristics e.g. production of sperm and semen, the change in voice, development of muscles, bones and male pattern hair growth.

The functions of the endocrine system ensure that the changing needs of the body are met in terms of homeostasis, growth and sexual development.

- Homeostasis is the maintenance of a constant state e.g. body temperature, mineral balance, blood pressure, fluid balance etc.
- Growth occurs in natural phases throughout life with rapid growth in the first year of life, slow, steady growth during childhood, rapid growth during puberty with growth ceasing at the average age of 16–17.
- Sexual development occurs in stages throughout life starting with puberty in both sexes and ending with menopause in females and andropause in males.

These functions are controlled, communicated and maintained by the links between the nervous and endocrine systems.

The nervous tissue of the hypothalamus in the brain provides the link between the nervous and endocrine systems. It forms an attachment with the pituitary gland allowing two-way communication to take place between the systems.

The hypothalamus receives information from the body through its nerve connections in the cerebrum of the brain. This stimulates the production of releasing hormones in the hypothalamus which regulate the hormone secretion of the pituitary gland. As a result the pituitary gland then produces hormones which control the other endocrine glands. The brain provides additional methods of stimulating hormone production in other endocrine glands by alerting the appropriate glands to changes in the internal and external environment e.g. the islets of Langerhans in the pancreas are alerted to the changes in blood sugar levels and the adrenal medulla is stimulated by stressful situations.

Reflexology can help to maintain balance between the endocrine and nervous systems, aiding function and efficiency. This is of particular benefit during times of unease with the systems due to and/or resulting in stress.

System sorter

ENDOCRINE SYSTEM

Nervous system

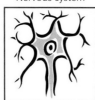

The hypothalamus and the pituitary gland link the nervous system with the endocrine system. A pituitary stalk joins the two structures in the brain. The hypothalamus secretes releasing hormones which activate the pituitary gland into producing hormones that affect the other glands.

Circulatory system

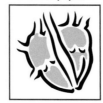

Hormones are suspended within blood plasma and are transported from the endocrine glands to the target cells of the body systems by the blood. Used hormones are transported by the blood to the kidneys for excretion.

Integumentary system

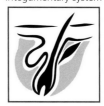

The production of melanin in the skin is stimulated by the hormone MSH (melanocyte stimulating hormone). MSH is produced in the anterior lobe of the pituitary gland and affects the colour of the skin.

Immune system

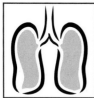

The thymus gland contributes to the immune functions of the body, producing T lymphocytes which help in the protection of the body against antigens.

Skeletal/muscular systems

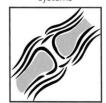

Adrenalin, secreted by the adrenal glands in response to stress, stimulates the flow of blood to the muscles in order to activate the body in preparation for fight or flight.

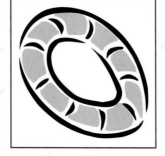

Adrenalin is the stress hormone responsible for the increase in breathing that takes place as a result of extreme emotions such as fear, anger, surprise etc.

The production of the hormones insulin and glucagon in the pancreas by the Islets of Langerhans helps to regulate blood sugar levels. The sugar present in the blood is processed from the food we eat by the digestive system.

Respiratory system

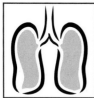

The anti-diuretic hormone vasopressin helps to regulate the body's fluid balance by distributing water to the vital cells and decreasing urine production in the kidneys.

Endocrine glands are made from epithelial tissue and secrete substances, in the form of hormones, directly into the blood.

If fluid balance is not controlled efficiently by the endocrine system, the lymphatic system suffers. Too little water inhibits the functions of the system preventing the free flow of lymph and elimination of toxins.

Digestive system

Genito-urinary system

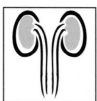

Cells

Lymphatic system

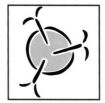

Consultation considerations

Changing hormone levels can have an effect on every aspect of the body and mind and certain considerations should be made during the consultation process to ensure that both the client and practitioner feel confident that the treatment will be suitable.

Oral

Questions relating to specific disorders of the endocrine system and the under-, over- or erratic production of hormones should be considered. In addition it is useful to ask a client how they are affected by their symptoms and how they manage them. This provides an insight into the types of coping mechanism they rely on. It may be that suggesting an alternative method of managing a condition such as the menopause provides the client with more relief than their current methods. Self-help provides a positive means to many stress related disorders.

Visual

Dysfunction of certain endocrine glands may be seen in physical symptoms:

- Imbalance of growth hormone in the pituitary gland can result in a gradual enlargement of the hands, feet and bones of the head and chest – a condition known as acromegaly.
- Increased appearance of facial and body hair in females known as hirsutism may result from an imbalance in prolactin in the pituitary gland and/or an excess of corticoids in the adrenal cortex.
- An imbalance of melanocyte stimulating hormone in the pituitary gland can cause chloasma (increased pigmentation) when too much is produced and vitiligo (decrease in pimentation) when not enough is being produced.
- Too much vasopressin in the system from the pituitary gland can cause oedema (swelling).
- Under- or overactive thyroid activity and differing levels of the production of thyroxine can result in excessive weight gain (underactive) or weight loss (overactive).

A visual analysis will help to piece together the signs and symptoms with the possible causes.

Aural

The complexity of the endocrine system can lead to much confusion in determining what is going on within the body, and care should be taken to listen carefully to all that is being said by the client. Make notes that can be easily read at a later date to help you to piece together the signs and symptoms. Do not make rash judgements and remember *never* to diagnose. Any one physical or psychological symptom may alert you to many of the body systems. Listen to all that is being said by the client and use the answers that are given as a springboard for further questions for the future. It is not necessary to ask all the questions in one consultation. The process is a progressive one that should be handled with care.

Olfactory

By linking the sense of smell with the other related skills it is possible to provide a balanced and thorough consultation, ensuring that careful consideration has been given to all relevant areas. Certain situations will warrant the use of only some of the consultation skills mentioned and others will call upon the use of all of them. A thorough consultation relies on the adaptation of such skills to meet the needs of each individual client.

Perceptive

It sometimes happens that one gets a sense of a person and what is going on within their body. This tends to happen when we open our minds and try *not* to analyse too deeply. All too often we get confused by what the body appears to be saying through other means as we search for an explanation that satisfies our left brain! Adopting an open mind frees the right brain into taking part in the search, often resulting in more creative and intuitive responses. This helps us get to know something without always having to question why, which in turn leads to a greater sense of awareness and possibly greater understanding.

Tactile

The endocrine glands are small in comparison with many other structures in the body and are often quite deep-seated e.g. pituitary and pineal in the brain. As a result it can be difficult to locate them when working over the reflexes. Sensitivity in the fingers and thumb and imagining that the tip is like a very small eye will help detect any localised stress. Touch stimulates the nerve endings in both the giver and the receiver. Frequent use of the art of touch helps to increase nerve stimulation.

Contraindication considerations

Clients with conditions relating to the endocrine system that require ongoing medical attention and medication, e.g. diabetes, should seek medical advice prior to the treatment. Reflexology is very effective at balancing the system which may in time lead to a gradual reduction of medication. However, this cannot be considered without ongoing medical advice.

Reflexes

The reflexes for the endocrine system are tiny and often deep-seated e.g. pituitary and pineal glands situated within the brain. Working over the whole of the feet, hands and ears ensures general treatment of these reflexes helping to balance their links with the other systems of the body. Specific treatment can be used as an aid to hormonal imbalance, the most common of which is stress-induced.

Tip

Some of the endocrine reflexes are treated as part of other systems e.g. the pancreas with the digestive system and the ovaries/testes with the genito-urinary system and as such do not necessarily need to be worked again. However, it is important to be aware of their dual functions in order to understand the associations with any possible imbalances.

The position of the reflexes

- Pituitary gland – mid point of the plantar/palmar aspect of the big toe/thumb and the antitragus of the ear.
- Pineal gland – upper section of the medial aspect of the big toe/thumb and the antitragus of the ear.
- Thyroid / parathyroid glands – lower, medial section of the dorsal aspect of the big toe/thumb. There is no specific reflex on the ear but working the throat reflex will affect these glands.
- Thymus gland – at the start of the thoracic vertebrae on the lateral edge of the foot/hand and the antihelix of the ear.
- Adrenal glands – zone 2 of the foot/hand above the reflex for the kidney and the tragus of the ear.
- Islets of Langerhans – pancreas reflex which is treated when working the digestive system and as such does not necessarily need further attention (see Chapter 16).
- Ovaries/testes – treated when working the genito-urinary system (see Chapter 17).

Endocrine system – order of work

Remember

The Islets of Langerhans in the pancreas and the ovaries and testes have been included in the order of work for the digestive and genito-urinary systems respectively.

Suggested order of work – feet

- *Pituitary gland* – place the thumb pad in the centre of the pad of the big toe pointing towards the top of the toe. Hook-in-and-back-up.
- *Pineal gland* – using the index finger, circle over the area at the top medial edge of the big toe close to the top corner of the nail.
- *Thyroid/parathyroid glands* – using the index finger placed at the base of the medial, dorsal aspect of the big toe, circle over the area for the thyroid and rock over the same area for the parathyroid.
- *Thymus gland* – slide the thumb down the medial edge of the foot to the start of the thoracic reflex point. Hook-in-and-back-up.
- *Adrenal glands* – slide thumb down the plantar aspect of the foot starting between the first two toes to just above waistline. Hook-in-and-back-up.

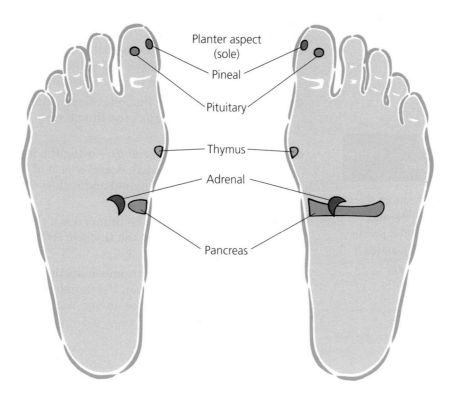

Planter aspect (sole)

Pineal

Pituitary

Thymus

Adrenal

Pancreas

Right foot

Left foot

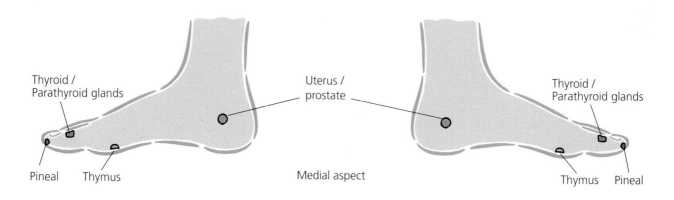

Thyroid / Parathyroid glands

Pineal

Thymus

Uterus / prostate

Medial aspect

Thyroid / Parathyroid glands

Thymus

Pineal

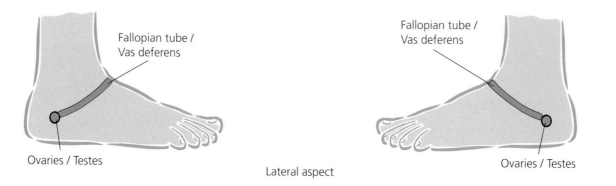

Fallopian tube / Vas deferens

Ovaries / Testes

Fallopian tube / Vas deferens

Ovaries / Testes

Lateral aspect

Remember

The Islets of Langerhans in the pancreas and the ovaries and testes have been included in the order of work for the digestive system and genito-urinary system respectively.

Suggested order of work – hands

- *Pituitary gland* – place the pad of the thumb or index finger in the centre of the pad of the thumb pointing towards the top of the thumb. Hook-in-and-back-up.
- *Pineal gland* – using the index finger, circle over the area at the top medial edge of the thumb close to the top corner of the nail.
- *Thyroid/parathyroid glands* – using the index finger placed at the base of the medial, dorsal aspect of the thumb, circle over the area for the thyroid and rock over the area for the parathyroid.
- *Thymus gland* – slide the thumb down the medial edge of the hand to the start of the thoracic reflex point. Hook-in-and-back-up.
- *Adrenal glands* – slide thumb down the palmar aspect of the hand starting between the thumb and index finger to just above waistline. Hook-in-and-back-up.

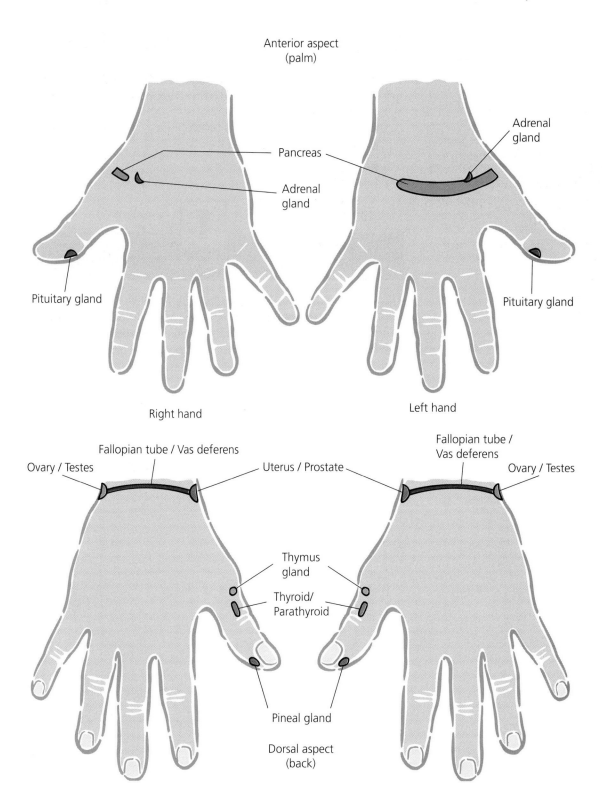

Anterior aspect
(palm)

Adrenal
gland

Pancreas

Adrenal
gland

Pituitary gland

Pituitary gland

Right hand

Left hand

Fallopian tube / Vas deferens

Fallopian tube /
Vas deferens

Ovary / Testes

Uterus / Prostate

Ovary / Testes

Thymus
gland

Thyroid/
Parathyroid

Pineal gland

Dorsal aspect
(back)

Tip

The pituitary and pineal glands share the same reflex point because of their position within the brain.

Suggested order of work – ears

Using the thumb to support the back of the ear apply small pressure movements to the specific reflex points:

- Pituitary and pineal – brain point
- Thymus gland
- Adrenal glands.

Remember

The thyroid and parathyroid glands are included in the treatment of the throat in the respiratory system (Chapter 15) order of work, the pancreas in the digestive system (Chapter 16) order of work and the ovaries/testes in the genito-urinary (Chapter 17) order of work. These reflexes do not necessarily need to be worked again.

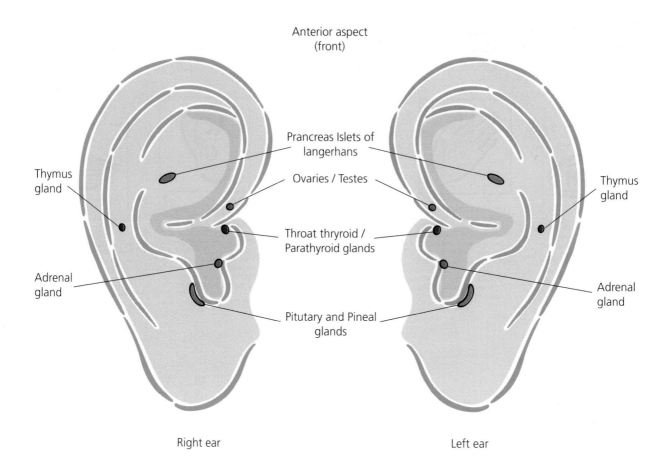

Anterior aspect
(front)

Prancreas Islets of
langerhans

Ovaries / Testes

Thymus
gland

Throat thryroid /
Parathyroid glands

Adrenal
gland

Pitutary and Pineal
glands

Thymus
gland

Adrenal
gland

Right ear

Left ear

Treatment tracker

ENDOCRINE SYSTEM

Visualisation

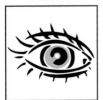

The endocrine system has a controlling action over the body which is slow to activate yet has long-lasting effects e.g. growth, puberty, menopause etc. Using a visual image can provide a positive impact on the balance of the controlling forces (hormones) when these major changes are taking place. Visualising a calm and peaceful place in which one feels safe and cherished surrounded by warmth and loving care helps to prepare the body and mind for the acceptance of such changes. The use of colour to accentuate the visualisation can add another dimension in the rebalancing of the endocrine system. Try to visualise the whole body bathing in the colours of the rainbow. If any of the colours lose their brightness or are difficult to imagine, try to visualise a bright white light infusing the rainbow with brightness.

Hands

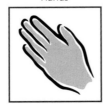

The endocrine system is located along the length of the hands and mirrored in the position of the chakras along the skull and spine. The reflex points for the individual glands are often deep-seated and difficult to locate and require the careful use of hook-in and back-up techniques.

Feet

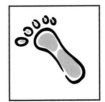

The endocrine system is located along the length of the feet and mirrored in the position of the chakras along the skull and spine. Imagining the chakras and their associated endocrine glands when working over the spinal reflexes helps to balance this system as well as strengthen its links with the nervous system.

Ears

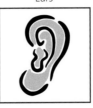

The endocrine system is located along the concha and lobes of the ears and mirrored in the position of the chakras along the skull and spine. The piercing of ears may be contributory to blockage of energy in certain reflex points and gentle, regular palpation to the whole ear can help to rebalance this energy flow.

Affirmation

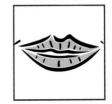

Throughout life activity within the endocrine system is varied in balance and action. Positive thought can provide a further balancing action on the system and the parts of the body it is controlling. Feeling that we have in some sense an element of control over our own bodies empowers us to achieve beyond the expected and is a strong force behind the ability to cope against adversity.

People often view change as being the end of something e.g. puberty is the end of childhood; menopause is the end of childbearing etc. A useful affirmation aims to turn a negative view into a positive view – 'I am entering a new and exciting phase of my life in which I am able to develop and prosper.'

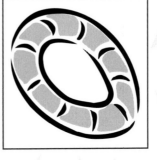

Each chakra corresponds with an individual endocrine gland, having an effect on its well-being.

- The first chakra is associated with the adrenal glands and the adaptation of the body in its quest for survival.
- The second chakra is associated with the ovaries in females and testes in males and in creative reproduction.
- The third chakra is associated with the pancreas and development through regulation and metabolism.
- The fourth chakra is associated with the thymus gland and physical and emotional protection.
- The fifth chakra is associated with the thyroid and parathyroid glands and physical and emotional growth.
- The sixth and seventh chakras are associated with the pineal and pituitary glands and the functions of clairvoyance, intuition and higher thinking.

The note D is linked with the endocrine system generally, although specific notes are associated with each endocrine gland:

- Adrenal glands – C and the mantra Lam.
- Ovaries/testes – D and the mantra Vam.
- Islets of Langerhans in the pancreas – E and the mantra Ram.
- Thymus gland – F and the mantra Yam.
- Thyroid/parathyroid glands – G and the mantra Ham.
- Pineal and pituitary glands – A and H and the mantras Ksham and Om.

In addition, the use of silence plays an important role in the balancing of this system. Listening to the sound of silence helps to create an opening for confusion to leave the body and harmony to enter.

Blue is linked with the endocrine system generally, although specific endocrine glands have an associated colour:

- Adrenal glands – red.
- Ovaries/testes – orange.
- Islets of Langerhans in the pancreas – yellow.
- Thymus gland – green.
- Thyroid/parathyroid glands – blue.
- Pituitary and pineal glands – indigo and violet.

The endocrine system is represented in each of the transverse zones and between zones 1–4 longitudinally. In addition, each endocrine gland is represented by a chakra which in turn are represented along the spinal reflex in zone 1 of the hands and feet. Working the zones and/or the specific reflex points offers an effective treatment of this system. Care should be taken when treating these reflexes to avoid overstimulation.

The triple burner meridian starts on the back of the ring finger, ascends the arm, neck and head and ends at the outer corner of the eye. It is naturally stimulated between 9 p.m.–11 p.m. and naturally calmed between 9 a.m.–11 a.m. The triple burner is a yang meridian and is coupled with the yin pericardium meridian. Their associated element is fire and their main functions include regulation and control of the body.

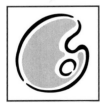

Colour

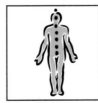

Chakras

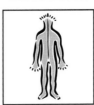

Zones

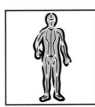

Meridians

Sound

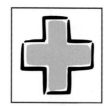

Activity

Pick six of the conditions listed and research them in greater depth. Check the indirect reflexes and add to them where relevant.

Common conditions

A detailed consultation is needed when considering the signs and symptoms relating to the endocrine system in order to determine the possible specific reflex that may be under excessive stress. The direct reflex will be the specific gland that is experiencing under- or over-activity. However, this will always have a knock-on effect on virtually every other part of the body. Endocrine glands secrete their hormones into the blood supply to be picked up by special target cells. These in turn initiate the appropriate responses. When this process malfunctions through either under- or over-activity within the glands, the rest of the body suffers the possible repercussions as excess pressure may be exerted on certain systems to compensate. Indirect reflexes are therefore far reaching and only the most obvious have been included in the list below.

An A–Z of common conditions associated with the endocrine system

- ACROMEGALY – an over secretion of the growth hormone GH in the anterior pituitary gland in adults can result in a thickening of skin and an enlargement of the hands, feet and face, particularly the lower jaw. *Direct reflex* = the pituitary gland. *Indirect reflexes* = hypothalamus, affected parts.
- ADDISON'S DISEASE – disorder of the adrenal glands. There is an underproduction of the hormones aldosterone and cortisol causing problems with metabolism and development. Muscle weakness, irregular menstrual cycle and dehydration are common symptoms. *Direct reflex* = the adrenal glands. *Indirect reflexes* = hypothalamus, pituitary gland, joints, ovaries.
- CHLOASMA – dark patches of skin which may appear as a result of a hypersecretion of MSH in the anterior pituitary gland. *Direct reflex* = the pituitary gland. *Indirect reflexes* = hypothalamus.
- CONN'S SYNDROME – results from the oversecretion of aldosterone in the adrenal cortex, leading to high blood pressure due to high potassium levels in the blood. Kidney failure may develop. *Direct reflex* = the adrenal glands. *Indirect reflexes* = hypothalamus, pituitary gland, kidneys.
- CRANIAL DIABETES INSIPIDUS – an inability of the body to conserve water due to hyposecretion of ADH in the posterior pituitary gland. *Direct reflex* = the kidneys. *Indirect reflexes* = hypothalamus, pituitary gland, all body systems.
- CRETINISM – see hypothyroidism.

- CUSHING'S SYNDROME – disorder of the adrenal glands. There is an overproduction of the hormones aldosterone and cortisol causing the opposite effects of Addison's disease. *Direct reflex* = the adrenal glands. *Indirect reflexes* = hypothalamus, pituitary gland.

- DIABETES – there are two types of diabetes, type one and type two, both resulting in increased levels of sugar in the blood. Type one, insulin-dependent diabetes, occurs when there is a hyposecretion of the hormone insulin produced in the Islets of Langerhans in the pancreas. Type two, maturity onset diabetes, occurs when the tissues are unable to respond to the secretion of insulin. Type one develops at an early age and requires regular injections of insulin, while type two develops at a later age and can usually be controlled by changes in diet. *Direct reflex* = the pancreas. *Indirect reflexes* = small and large intestines, liver, kidneys.

- DWARFISM – undersecretion of growth hormone GH from the anterior pituitary gland during childhood results in the failure of bones and organs to grow to normal size. *Direct reflex* = the pituitary gland. *Indirect reflexes* = hypothalamus, affected organs.

- GALACTORRHOEA – an excess of milk flow caused by an over secretion of prolactin in the anterior pituitary gland. *Direct reflex* = the pituitary gland. *Indirect reflexes* = hypothalamus, breasts, axillary lymph nodes.

- GIGANTISM – oversecretion of growth hormone GH from the anterior pituitary gland during childhood results in an abnormal development in the length of long bones. *Direct reflex* = the pituitary gland. *Indirect reflexes* = hypothalamus, joints.

- GOITRE – enlargement of the thyroid gland caused by a lack of iodine. *Direct reflex* = the thyroid gland. *Indirect reflexes* = pituitary gland, hypothalamus, throat.

- GRAVES' DISEASE – see hyperthyroidism.

- GYNAECOMASTIA – overproduction of oestrogen in males causing the development of the breasts. *Direct reflex* = the testes. *Indirect reflexes* = pituitary gland, hypothalamus, breasts.

- HIRSUTISM – an overproduction of testosterone in females leading to the development of male pattern hair growth. Common times for this include puberty, pregnancy and menopause. *Direct reflex* = the ovaries. *Indirect reflexes* = hypothalamus, pituitary gland, adrenal glands, thyroid gland.

- HYPERCALCAEMIA – excess calcium in the blood caused by the oversecretion of parathormone in the parathyroid glands. *Direct reflex* = the parathyroid glands. *Indirect reflexes* = the thyroid gland.

- HYPERGLYCAEMIA – undersecretion of insulin and/or oversecretion of glucagons in the pancreas causing high blood sugar levels. *Direct reflexes* = the pancreas. *Indirect reflexes* = small and large intestines.

- HYPERTHYROIDISM – overactive thyroid production of the hormone thyroxine causing the metabolism to speed up resulting in loss of weight, increased heart rate and swelling of the tissue behind the eyes. The eyes develop a prominent bulge. Hyperthyroidism is also known as GRAVES' DISEASE and THYROTOXICOSIS. *Direct reflex* = the thyroid gland. *Indirect reflexes* = hypothalamus, pituitary gland, small and large intestines, eyes.

- HYPOCALCAEMIA – lack of calcium in the blood caused by the undersecretion of parathormone in the parathyroid glands. *Direct reflex* = the parathyroid glands. *Indirect reflexes* = thyroid glands.

- HYPOGLYCAEMIA – an overproduction of insulin causes low blood sugar levels with symptoms similar to drunkenness e.g. blurred vision, sweating, trembles and a lack of concentration. This condition may accompany diabetes. *Direct reflex* = the pancreas. *Indirect reflexes* = small and large intestines, eyes.

- HYPOTHYROIDISM – underactive thyroid production of the hormone thyroxine causing the metabolism to slow down resulting in weight gain. Hypothyroidism at birth results in the disorder CRETINISM and in adults MYXOEDEMA if untreated. The body systems work at a slower than normal pace. *Direct reflex* = the thyroid gland. *Indirect reflexes* = hypothalamus, pituitary gland.

- HYPER PARATHYROIDISM – overproduction of the hormone parathormone from the parathyroid glands causes a decrease in calcium in the bones. This may lead to osteoporosis, where the bones become very brittle. *Direct reflex* = the parathyroid glands. *Indirect reflexes* = thyroid gland, joints.

- HYPO PARATHYROIDISM – underproduction of the hormone parathormone from the parathyroid glands causing a decrease of calcium in the body. *Direct reflex* = the parathyroid glands. *Indirect reflexes* = thyroid gland, joints.

- MYXOEDEMA – see hypothyroidism.

- POLYCYSTIC OVARIAN SYNDROME – underproduction of LH in females resulting in the development of ovarian cysts. This is accompanied by an irregular menstrual cycle and sometimes infertility. *Direct reflex* = the pituitary gland. *Indirect reflexes* = hypothalamus, ovaries.

- SAD (seasonal affective disorder) – an overproduction of the hormone melatonin produced in the pineal gland. The result is depression and lethargy especially during the winter months. *Direct reflex* = the pineal gland. *Indirect reflexes* = ovaries/testes.

- STRESS – prolonged negative stress results in long term overproduction of the hormones cortisol and adrenalin from the adrenal glands. This causes overstimulation of some body systems e.g. muscles and under stimulation of other body systems e.g. digestion which results in aching muscles and poor digestion. *Direct reflex* = the adrenal glands. *Indirect reflexes* = hypothalamus, pituitary gland, stomach, small and large intestines, kidneys, joints, lymph nodes.

- TETANY – abnormally low levels of calcium in the blood causing muscle spasms mainly in the hands, feet and face. May be caused by an under production of parathormone. *Direct reflex* = the parathyroid glands. *Indirect reflexes* = thyroid gland, joints, face.

- THYROTOXICOSIS – hyperthyroidism caused by the overproduction of thyroxine. *Direct reflex* = the thyroid gland. *Indirect reflexes* = hypothalamus, pituitary gland.

- VIRILISM – an overproduction of testosterone in females causing the onset of male characteristics including receding hair line, increased body and facial hair and the deepening of the voice. The menstrual cycle is also affected. *Direct reflexes* = the ovaries. *Indirect reflexes* = hypothalamus, pituitary gland, fallopian tubes, uterus.

- VITILIGO – white patches of skin that may be caused by an undersecretion of MSH in the anterior pituitary gland. *Direct reflex* = the pituitary gland. *Indirect reflexes* = the hypothalamus.

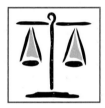

Holistic harmony

The endocrine system is constantly alert and ready for action, providing spurts of activity at certain times in order to promote the healthy development and maintenance of the human body throughout life. As such, it requires internal balance and harmony in order to create the balance and harmony required in the body as a whole.

Air

Research has found that many synthetic chemicals have a harmful effect on the well-being of the endocrine system. These harmful chemicals are often inhaled through the air breathed into the body and care should be taken to avoid the use of pollutants both personally and globally. Some pollutants have been found to initiate changes in metabolism, growth and development, fertility and even emotions because of their effects on the endocrine system.

The use of essential oils in aromatherapy can have a balancing effect on the endocrine system, as many act as hormone harmonisers. The inhalation of certain essential oils can stimulate the production of hormones or mimic the action of certain hormones.

Water

The balance of water within the body is controlled by the links between the nervous and endocrine systems. The nervous system picks up on the internal need for water and the endocrine system alerts the other body systems to methods of conserving water. The posterior lobe of the pituitary gland secretes the antidiuretic hormone vasopressin, which helps to regulate the flow of water into some of the cells of the body as well as decrease the production of urine in the kidneys. Vital cells of the body contain vasopressin receptors which ensure that water is received to maintain the function of these cells. Vasopressin is involved in the rationing and distribution of water when the body is suffering from dehydration, directing the water to the most vital cells.

Alcohol and caffeine suppress the secretion of vasopressin which leads to general dehydration. To cope with this situation, endorphins are produced by the body which contribute to the addictive effects of alcohol and caffeine. Women have a natural tendency to produce more endorphins and as such appear to become addicted to alcohol and caffeine more readily than men.

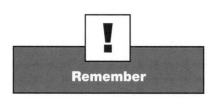

Remember

Endorphins are neurotransmitters associated with raising the pain threshold.

Nutrition

Hormones are produced from components of the food we eat. The majority of hormones are protein-based except for steroids e.g. corticoids produced in the adrenal cortex, which are fat-based. In turn hormones help to regulate the use of nutrients taken into the body by maintaining the correct balance e.g. fluid, minerals etc. As demands on the body and within the body change, so does the secretion of hormones. As a result, a healthy diet is a contributory factor in the well-being of the endocrine system. Just as pollutants in the air affect the functioning of this system, so do pollutants in the food we eat. Fresh, organic foods offer a more effective solution in the healthy functioning of this system and the whole body than over-processed, chemically enhanced or modified foods.

Age

The passing of time brings with it vital changes in the body activated by the endocrine system. From the effects of puberty, menstruation, pregnancy and menopause, women have more radical changes affecting their bodies than men do in the same space of time. However, any changes bring about physical and psychological pressures that both men and women can find difficult to cope with. Not only do we have to cope with the ageing process in ourselves but also that in our loved ones. Many of those changes are irreversible without the intervention of medical procedures e.g. face lifts etc. Even then, they are only able to make superficial changes, they cannot reverse the effect the passing of time has had on our body, mind and spirit as a whole.

Ageing brings with it a gradual slowing down of functions of the body, which like any machine needs careful handling the older it gets. Adaptations to life style are needed, and it becomes even more important to pick up on the many signs the body gives out everyday expressing its changing needs and desires.

Rest

Stress activates the endocrine system. Long-term stress exerts excessive strain on the system, reducing its effectiveness at maintaining homeostasis. As a result, functions such as maintenance of fluid and mineral balance, metabolism and sexual development etc. may be adversely affected. The endocrine system, like the rest of the body, can deal effectively with short, sharp bursts of stress which should then be followed by periods of rest in order to counteract the effects.

Relaxation techniques, used daily, help to counteract the potentially debilitating effects of the stresses associated with everyday living and can be experienced through meditation, breathing exercises, self-massage, affirmations and visualisations etc.

Activity

Movement ensures effective transportation of hormones through increased blood flow. This is an important factor in the distribution of hormones from the endocrine glands to the target cells of each system as well as strengthening the links between the nervous and endocrine systems.

Good posture also contributes to the well-being of the endocrine glands in relation to their position within the body. Maintaining the natural shape of the spine without placing any undue stress on specific parts will be of direct benefit to these glands.

Combining periods of stress-free activity with relaxation are an ideal way of rebalancing the daily effects of stress and these can be gained through activities such as yoga and pilates which include controlled movement and breathing with positive thinking.

Awareness

Many clients seek reflexology for the treatment of menstrual problems. Having an awareness of the process surrounding the monthly cycle is useful in the treatment of female clients.

The menstrual cycle lasts for approximately 28 days and is controlled by the hypothalamus which stimulates the production of FSH and LH in the anterior lobe of the pituitary gland. There are three distinct phases associated with the menstrual cycle:

1. Menstrual phase – if an ovum is not fertilised the lining of the uterus breaks down and bleeding occurs, lasting approximately five days.
2. Proliferative phase – hormones stimulate the lining of the uterus. This process takes approximately nine days at which time a new ovum is released from a follicle in one of the ovaries and passes along the fallopian tube to the uterus. This is known as ovulation.
3. Secretory stage – hormones stimulate the renewal of the lining of the uterus, the retention of fluid and the production of

mucus in preparation for entry by a sperm and fertilisation of the ovum to take place. This process takes approximately fourteen days. If fertilisation does not occur then the whole cycle begins again.

Pregnancy occurs when fertilisation is successful and the ovum becomes embedded in the wall of the uterus. The production of the hormone HCG (human chorionic gonadotrophin) takes place which maintains the lining of the uterus, preventing menstruation and the production of new ova.

Menopause marks the end of childbearing years in women as changes in hormone levels take place. The menstrual cycle becomes irregular and eventually stops all together. Menopause is often accompanied by short-term flushing and sweating, loss of bone mass, loss of pubic and axillary hair, thinning of skin and mood swings.

Special care

As a race, our obsession with appearance is legendary. Every culture throughout history has paid enormous amounts of attention to the way in which its people are portrayed externally and it appears none more so than now. And it is the endocrine system that is responsible for the changes in our appearance that we sometimes find very difficult to cope with. The endocrine system controls growth and sexual development initiating puberty and menopause/andropause.

- The onset of puberty in girls occurs when they reach approximately seven-and-a-half stone in weight. In recent years the age when girls start their periods has come down significantly in line with the significant increases in weight at an earlier age.
- An early onset of puberty often signifies an earlier onset of menopause.
- Weight gain is synonymous with menopause as the shift in hormone balance from female to male encourages the tendency to store fat around the waist.
- An underactive thyroid gland is contributory to weight gain as the production of the hormone thyroxine regulates the amount of energy the body burns.
- The adrenal cortex is responsible for producing cortisol in response to stress which boosts sugar levels in the blood. As a result the Islets of Langerhans secrete insulin to reduce blood sugar levels. It has been found that insulin encourages the body to store more fat.

A healthy body and mind relies on acceptance of the passing stages of life and an awareness of the ways in which special care can help to alleviate the associated problems. Complementary therapies offer a means to special care that is holistic in its approach, natural in its function and positive in its result.

Case study

The endocrine system has a controlling effect on all aspects of a person's physical, psychological and spiritual well-being and as such is a focus for the treatment of many disorders. It is often difficult to interpret how and why a particular endocrine gland affects the body as whole and indeed the reasons why a particular endocrine gland is tender during treatment. It is therefore important to have a period of reflection post-treatment in order to help to clear things up in your own mind. It is useful to have access to a selection of medical books to which to refer when further explanation is needed e.g. nurse's dictionary, directory of prescribed drugs and their possible side effects, anatomy and physiology books etc. In addition, health and fitness magazines, holistic journals etc. provide an excellent source of updated material which is often of benefit when trying to understand the endocrine system.

An increasing amount of male clients are joining women in seeking reflexology treatment as a result of hormonal imbalance, of which stress is perhaps the largest factor. In addition to the effects of puberty on the male and female body, the medical profession are beginning to acknowledge the change in hormone levels as a man reaches middle age and the emergence of the male menopause or andropause as a medical condition is testament to this. Reflexology provides a practical and positive means to help to counterbalance the physical, psychological and spiritual effects of such times in a person's life. The effects of disturbed hormone activity in the testes in men and ovaries in women leads to a number of symptoms that are further aggravated by the secretion of stress hormones from the adrenal glands.

The reflex points of the endocrine glands are often deep-seated and difficult to locate because of their position in the body and relative size. Treating the system after most of the systems have been worked ensures greater access as the body is relaxed and warm. The body and thus the endocrine glands are more open to treatment and become more responsive as a result. Treatment of the endocrine system relies heavily on knowledge, skill and intuition and is perhaps the hardest system to understand at each level. If a gland is tender during treatment for reasons that are unclear it may be wise not to mention it to the client until you are sure that first of all you were in the right place, and second that there is an explanation that is justifiable, e.g. mentioning that a particular gland has come up during treatment without logical justification may be cause for alarm, which increases stress levels creating further imbalance. It is wise to keep a check on whether or not tenderness in a

▶

Case study (continued)

particular gland appears on a regular basis and explore the possible reasons/causes. Clients have a tendency to pick up on negative comments, e.g. 'your thyroid gland is tender but I don't know why – it's probably nothing'. The main focus will be thyroid, tender and probably. The possible interpretation being that the thyroid gland must be important, if it is tender there must be something wrong and it is probably serious! As a result of possible misinterpretation a person will feel far worse post-treatment that they did pre-treatment and will continue to do so until their mind is put at rest. It is therefore important to always consider the weight our words carry and take extreme care when giving feedback.

Task

Using the treatment card as a guide, work over the reflexes on the feet, hands or ears for the endocrine system noting down the tender areas. Begin with a consultation (new or updated), continue with relaxation movements and add in the treatment of the previous systems. Finish with relaxation movements, breathing exercises, feedback and aftercare advice.

Knowledge review

1   With which system is the endocrine system closely linked?

2   What is the name given to the master gland and why?

3   What does the hormone melatonin regulate and which gland is responsible for its secretion?

4   Which gland has a regulatory effect on the metabolism?

5   Which glands help to regulate the calcium and phosphorus levels in the body?

6   Which glands contribute to the fight or flight response?

7   Where is insulin produced and why?

8   Where are the thyroid and parathyroid reflexes located on the feet?

9   In which longitudinal and transverse zones are the adrenal glands located on the hands?

10   Where is the brain point located on the ears?

19

Reflexes of the lymphatic system

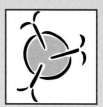

The lymphatic system is a one-way circulatory system that works in conjunction with the blood circulation. The lymphatic circulation is responsible for transporting unwanted substances away from the cells that the venous blood is unable to deal with. The fluid **lymph** flows through the lymphatic system which is comprised of **lymphatic vessels**, **nodes**, **tissue** and **ducts**.

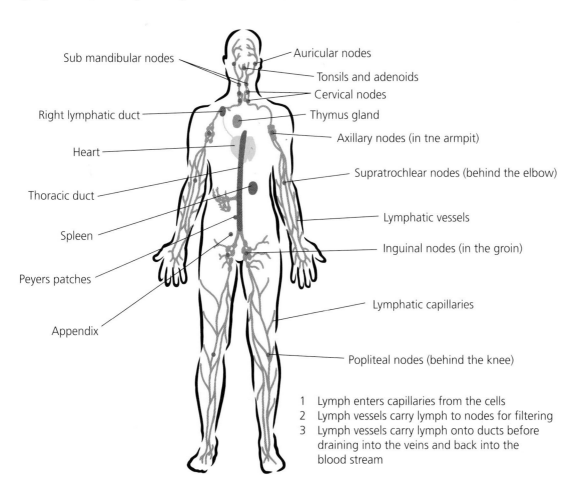

Sub mandibular nodes

Auricular nodes

Tonsils and adenoids

Cervical nodes

Right lymphatic duct

Thymus gland

Heart

Axillary nodes (in tne armpit)

Supratrochlear nodes (behind the elbow)

Thoracic duct

Lymphatic vessels

Spleen

Inguinal nodes (in the groin)

Peyers patches

Lymphatic capillaries

Appendix

Popliteal nodes (behind the knee)

1   Lymph enters capillaries from the cells
2   Lymph vessels carry lymph to nodes for filtering
3   Lymph vessels carry lymph onto ducts before draining into the veins and back into the blood stream

Lymphatic nodes, tissue and ducts

Lymph is a straw-coloured fluid similar to blood plasma which forms as a result of the blood passing substances into the interstitial fluid that bathes the cells.

Remember

Interstitial fluid forms a link between the blood and the cells, allowing oxygen and nutrients to pass into the cells from the blood and waste products such as carbon dioxide to pass back out.

Lymphatic vessels start as lymphatic capillaries which pick up lymph. They develop into larger tubes and follow the course of veins through the body.

Tip

Lymphatic vessels are similar to veins as they rely on the action of the skeletal muscles to aid flow and they contain valves to prevent back flow.

Lymphatic nodes – lymphatic vessels pass through nodes which are situated in strategic places around the body i.e. underarms, groin, neck, elbow, knee etc. where the lymph is filtered to remove and destroy unwanted and harmful substances (antigens). Nodes are also responsible for defending the body by producing antibodies in response to an antigen.

Lymphatic tissue forms additional structures in the body that help in the defence of the body including:

- The **spleen** – situated in the upper left hand side of the abdomen. The spleen is responsible for the removal of old, damaged and defective blood cells as well as being a reservoir for blood.

Fascinating Fact

Blood stored in the spleen can be diverted to other parts of the body when needed e.g. haemorrhage (excess bleeding).

- The **thymus gland** – an endocrine gland (see Chapter 18) which responds to antigens that invade the body by producing T-lymphocytes.
- **Tonsils**, **adenoids** and **appendix** – help to defend the body by destroying harmful invaders as part of the respiratory (Chapter 15) and digestive systems (Chapter 16).
- **Peyer's patches** – areas of lymphatic tissue situated in the latter part of the small intestine helping to prevent infection.

Fascinating Fact

Lymphatic tissue also forms **lacteals** in the small intestine. Lacteals are ducts which absorb digested fats.

Lymphatic ducts –filtered lymph is collected into two ducts, the thoracic and right lymphatic ducts, where it is drained into the veins.

- The thoracic duct is the main duct extending from the lumbar vertebrae to the base of the neck collecting lymph from the left side of the head, neck and thorax, the left arm, both legs as well as the abdomen and pelvic areas, draining into the left subclavian vein.
- The right lymphatic duct is situated in the base of the neck collecting lymph from the right side of the head, neck and thorax as well as the right arm, draining it into the right subclavian vein.

The lymphatic circulation has three main functions: circulation, transportation and defence.

- Circulation of lymph is one way – *away* from the cells.
- Lymphatic vessels are responsible for the transportation of waste products from the cells to the nodes and ducts for filtering and drainage into the bloodstream. Lacteals transport digested fats from the digestive system to the bloodstream.
- Lymph nodes and tissue provide a filtering system for lymph where macrophage cells engulf antigens and lymphocytes (white blood cells) produce antibodies in defence.

The lymphatic system is complementary to the blood circulatory system and together they help to regulate many of the body's vital functions, providing the force that links the systems of the body.

System sorter

LYMPHATIC SYSTEM

Nervous system

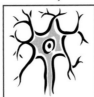

Circulatory system

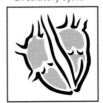

Integumentary system

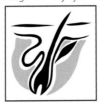

Skeletal/muscular systems

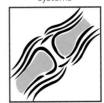

Immune system

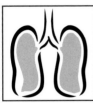

The effects of stress can seriously impair the immune responses in the lymphatic system. Long-term stress can have a debilitating effect on the lymphatic system leaving the body vulnerable to diseases and disorders.

The lymphatic system works closely with the blood circulation, collecting excessive tissue fluid and returning it to the bloodstream once the filtering process has been completed.

The skin, hair and nails contribute to the immune functions of the body by providing a first line of defence against external attack. This system helps to prevent the entry of pathogens into the body. (A pathogen is a disease-causing agent e.g. viruses, bacteria, fungi and parasites.)

The lymphatic system forms an important part of the immune system, helping to destroy pathogens in the event of entry into the body. Specialised lymphocytes recognise the invader and respond with a specific defence mechanism.

Action of the skeletal muscles encourages the flow of lymph through the system. Strategically placed valves within the lymphatic vessels prevent back flow of lymph. Lack of muscular action may cause localised oedema.

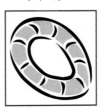

The respiratory system contributes to the removal of waste products from the body with the expulsion of carbon dioxide during expiration. Lymphatic cells are also present within the system to help to guard against pathogenic attack.

The digestive system is protected by the presence of lymphatic tissue. Peyer's patches are present in the mucous membrane of the lower part of the small intestine and the appendix projects from the caecum. Small lymphatic ducts called lacteals assist in the absorption of fats from the digestive system.

Cells called macrophages and lymphocytes are found within the lymphatic system and help to defend the body against attack. Macrophages are phagocytic cells that have the power to ingest cell debris and bacteria. Lymphocytes are white blood cells formed in lymphatic tissue that produce antibodies in response to antigens.

The kidneys help to control the volume of fluid within the body, including lymph. A lack of water results in inhibited lymph flow contributing to the problems associated with static lymph e.g. cellulite.

At times of invasion by a pathogen the body responds with the production of hormones. The thymus gland produces a group of hormones known as thymosins which stimulate the production of special T lymphocytes.

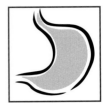

Digestive system

Respiratory system

Genito-urinary system

Endocrine system

Cells

Consultation considerations

In order to determine the stress levels of the lymphatic system it is useful to take note of the following considerations during the consultation, remembering that whilst it may not be possible to obtain all information during the first consultation, it is important to be aware of some necessary facts so that a safe treatment may be carried out.

Oral

Questions relating to the lymphatic system may include asking about the following:

- Swellings that may have occurred in areas of nodes e.g. neck, underarms and groin.
- Any problems past or present with adenoids, tonsils and appendix.

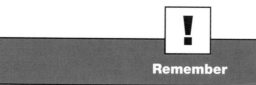

Remember

If a person has had any lymphatic structures removed, further questions should be asked with reference to date of surgery, any resulting medication and any further problems. Extra care should be taken over reflexes where recent operations have taken place. If in any doubt avoid the area or use gentle movements to soothe.

- Any problems with retention of water e.g. swollen ankles, cellulite.

Visual

The occurrence of any localised swelling in the tissues as a result of static lymph may be clearly seen in the ankles and lower legs. Cellulite may also be identified by a sluggish appearance to the skin with accompanying puffiness and dimpling, especially when the skin is pinched together. Further problems may also be evident in the condition of the facial skin. Static lymph often accompanies an acne skin type, sinus problems etc. A visual examination of the feet, hands and/or ears may confirm the presence of static lymph. These parts will appear puffy, especially in the region of the specific reflexes e.g. nodes and tissue.

Aural

Piecing together the answers a client gives to a variety of questions provides the practitioner with the ammunition needed to perform a safe and effective reflexology treatment. Active listening remains a vital component in ensuring that the information received is interpreted and used correctly for the benefit of each individual client. We should try to avoid making rash judgements because we are hearing what we want to hear and aim to use active listening as a means of understanding each individual client.

 Angel advice

We may be asking the same basic questions but we should not expect to hear the same replies.

Olfactory

Poor lymphatic function results in poor filtering and elimination of waste from the body and this may be picked up by our sense of smell.

It is also useful to be aware of the factors relating to the elimination of waste through the sweat glands. The regular consumption of certain foods e.g. herbs and spices may be picked up in the odour of sweat and breath e.g. garlic.

Perceptive

As with all processes associated with elimination, the body is required to physically let go in order for the function to be maintained. Psychological factors may impede the ability to let go as a person tries hard to keep emotions and feelings locked inside. This may have a knock-on effect on the physical functions, and it is useful to consider the links between body and mind to gain a truer insight into the workings of a human being. This is not something that may always be picked up during the first consultation and it may take many treatments before an awareness of the inner feelings demonstrate a manifestation of the physical symptoms, if at all. Developing our perceptive skills can be carried out by trying to open the mind, allowing us to make use of the interflow of the three main channels of energy – our personal energy, that of our client and the eternal energy that flows around us.

Tactile

By touching any areas of swelling, the practitioner can determine their nature. Oedema associated with static lymph will feel puffy to touch. Areas of cellulite may feel bumpy, similar to the feel of orange peel, and cold due to the poor blood circulation.

By touching the feet, hands and/or ears similar feelings will be detected and drainage movements of these parts play a vital contributory factor in restoring good function to the system as a whole.

Contraindication considerations

Extreme caution should be paid to disorders to the lymphatic system such as cancer, and treatment is not advisable without medical consent, approval and guidance. Some clients suffering with cancer decide not to continue with medical treatment, preferring to seek alternative treatment methods. If called upon to treat such a client with reflexology, a practitioner must be aware of their role in the possible progression of the disease and careful consideration should be taken prior to any treatment taking place.

Reflexes

The lymphatic system is complementary to the circulatory system and as such forms a part of the systemic systems highlighted in Chapter 13. General treatment ensures that this system is worked aiding lymphatic flow, transportation of waste and the body's defence mechanisms. It is of additional benefit to treat specific reflexes to aid these functions further, and if carried out towards the end of the treatment ensures improved elimination processes.

The position of the reflexes

The specific reflexes of the lymphatic system include:

- Tonsils and adenoids = treated as part of the respiratory system (Chapter 15) when working the throat.
- Thymus gland – treated when working the endocrine system (Chapter 17).
- Spleen – treated when working the digestive system (Chapter 16).
- Appendix – treated when working the digestive system (Chapter 16.
- Axillary nodes and breasts – dorsal aspect of the foot/hand over the thoracic reflex and the thoracic reflex of the ear.
- Inguinal nodes and groin – around the outer anklebone of the foot/hand and the hip reflex of the ear.
- Joints – along the lateral edge of the foot/hand and the antihelix of the ear.
- Spine – along the medial edge of the foot/hand and the medial edge of the antihelix of the ear.

Tip

There is a specific reflex point on the ears for the tonsils. They are located on the lower section of the lobe.

Lymphatic system – order of work

Tip

Drainage movements over the joints benefits the supratrochlear and popliteal nodes of the elbows and knees as well as drainage of the arms and legs generally.

Remember

The tonsils and adenoids have been included in the order of work for the respiratory system and the spleen and appendix have been included in the order of work for the digestive system. However, the order of work may be changed or rearranged to suit.

Suggested order of work – feet

- *Axillary nodes and breasts* – using the length of both thumbs, apply alternate draining movements to the dorsal aspect of the foot from the base of the toes to the diaphragm line.
- *Inguinal nodes and groin* – using the pads of the fingers, circle around the lateral and medial anklebones.
- *Joints* – using the pads of the fingers, circle up the lateral edge of the foot from the base to the top. Repeat twice more.
- *Spine* – using the pads of the fingers, circle up the medial edge of the foot from the base to the top. Repeat twice more.

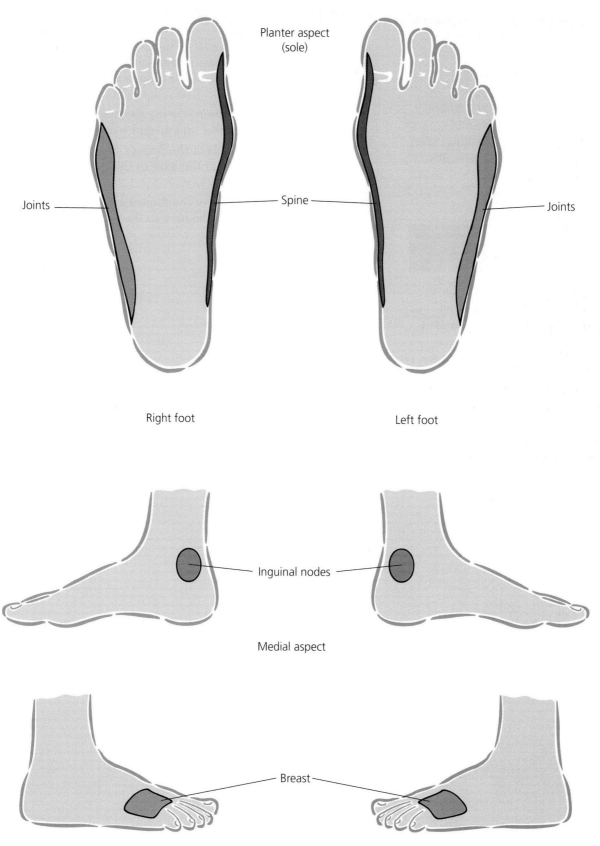

Planter aspect
(sole)

Joints ——— ——— Spine ——— ——— Joints

Right foot   Left foot

——— Inguinal nodes

Medial aspect

——— Breast ———

Lateral aspect

Tip

Drainage movements over the joints benefits the supratrochlear and popliteal nodes of the elbows and knees as well as drainage of the arms and legs generally.

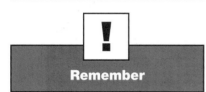

Remember

The tonsils and adenoids have been included in the order of work for the respiratory system and the spleen and appendix have been included in the order of work for the digestive system. However, the order of work may be changed or rearranged to suit.

Suggested order of work – hands

- *Axillary nodes and breasts* – using the length of the thumbs apply alternate drainage movements to the dorsal aspect of the hand from the base of the fingers to the diaphragm line.
- *Inguinal nodes and groin* – using the pads of the fingers circle around the lateral and medial wrist bones.
- *Joints* – using the pads of the fingers circle up the lateral aspect of the hand from the base to the top. Repeat twice more.
- *Spine* – using the pads of the fingers circle up the medial edge of the hand from the base to the top. Repeat twice more.

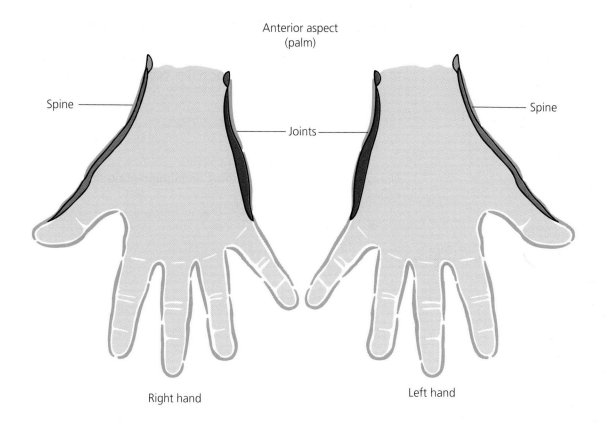

Anterior aspect
(palm)

Spine

Joints

Spine

Right hand

Left hand

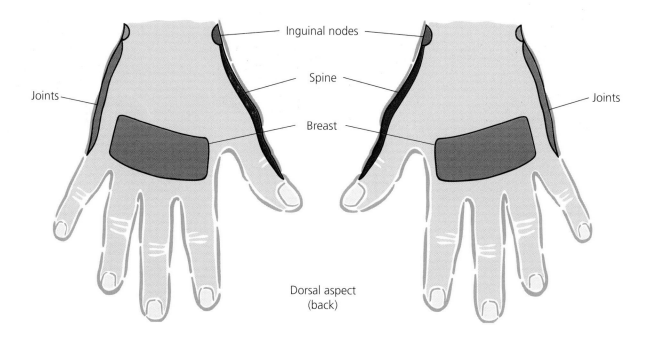

Inguinal nodes

Spine

Joints

Breast

Joints

Dorsal aspect
(back)

Suggested order of work – ears

With the thumb supporting the back of the ear use the index finger to apply pressure to the specific reflex points:

- Appendix
- Spleen
- Tonsils.

Using the index finger in sliding a sliding motion drain the specific reflex points:

- Spine
- Joints.

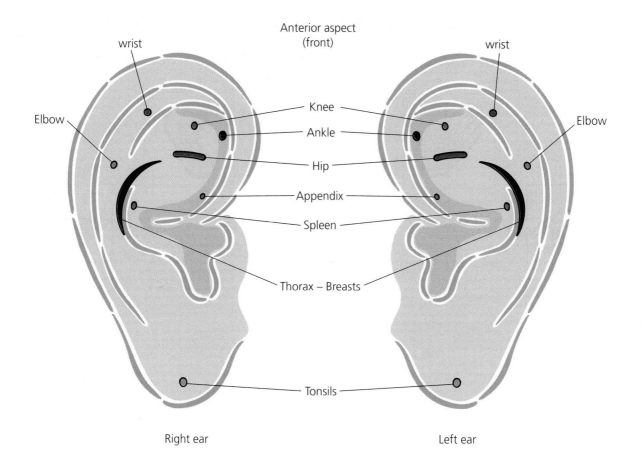

Anterior aspect
(front)

wrist

wrist

Elbow

Elbow

Knee

Ankle

Hip

Appendix

Spleen

Thorax – Breasts

Tonsils

Right ear

Left ear

Treatment tracker

LYMPHATIC SYSTEM

Hands

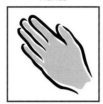

Feet

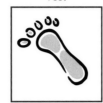

Ears

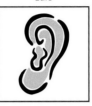

Visualisation

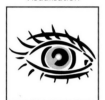

Affirmation

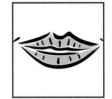

The lymphatic system is represented generally in all aspects of the hands and as such any form of treatment to the hand will be of benefit. Hand exercises contribute to the effectiveness of this system and may be incorporated into the aftercare advice given to a client. It may also be useful for the practitioner to practice hand exercises prior to giving a reflexology treatment to aid the overall performance of their hands.

The lymphatic system is represented generally in all aspects of the feet. Ending the reflexology treatment with lymphatic drainage movements to the feet and legs is an ideal way of completing the treatment, ensuring the effective drainage of the toxins released.

The lymphatic system is represented generally in all aspects of the ears. Self-treatment is a useful tool if applied to the ears to help speed up localised circulation. The helix of the ear has relatively poor circulation and it is for this reason that piercing of this area should be avoided. Poor circulation results in poor healing.

It is useful to try to imagine in our mind's eye the actions of the lymphatic system in protecting the body. Many people liken the lymphatic cells to minute soldiers silently protecting the body. These soldiers march en masse to the site of infection/invasion/disease etc. to exert their protective powers. Using the mind in this way helps to strengthen the immune functions of the body as well as provide a positive focal point. This theme can also be used to help to maintain a well body by visualising the soldiers constantly on guard and ready for action.

The lymphatic system helps to purify and refresh the body, assisting protection against disease and a useful affirmation is one which reinforces this: 'To be cleansed is to be refreshed. To be refreshed is to be purified. To be purified is to be alive – I am cleansed, purified and alive.'

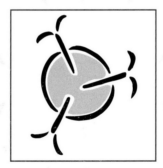

The colour green is linked with the lymphatic system. Green has a calming and balancing effect through its association with nature and new life and brings a freshness to the system. The yellow contained in green provides a purifying effect on the system and is associated with the elimination of waste. Plants and flowers add a different dimension to the use of colour and can enhance the effects. The addition of water can also help to magnify the cleansing process.

The note A is associated with the lymphatic system. Music that is flowing with good rhythm has a therapeutic effect, encouraging a rhythmical flow of lymph through the system. The flow of lymph is dependent solely on the flow of movement within the body and music can help to stimulate the natural body rhythms. Dancing is a brilliant exercise for all aspects of well-being and can be incorporated into the aftercare advice.

The second and fourth chakras have a specific effect on the lymphatic system:

- The fourth chakra is associated with the circulatory systems – of which the lymphatic system is a part – contributing to the protective functions of the system.
- The second chakra is associated with the liquids of the body, e.g. lymph, and their free flow through the body.

The systemic factors of the lymphatic system, the lymphatic vessels, are represented in all zones of the body with specific reflex points e.g. the spleen, appendix, adenoids and tonsils etc. according to their specific position in the body. Treating the general and specific lymphatic reflexes helps to strengthen the protection and self-preservation of body, mind and spirit.

The spleen meridian starts at the big toe, runs up the leg, bends into the pelvis, runs up the abdomen and ends in the shoulder. It is naturally stimulated between 9 a.m.–11 a.m. and naturally calmed between 9 p.m.–11 p.m. The yin spleen meridian is coupled with the yang stomach meridian and is said to rule 'transformation and transportation'. The element of the spleen and stomach meridians is earth.

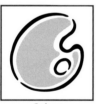

Colour

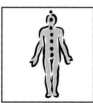

Chakras

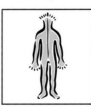

Zones

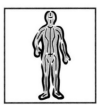

Meridians

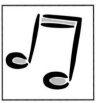

Sound

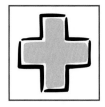

Common conditions

Because of its links with the immune functions of the body, the common conditions affecting the lymphatic system are listed in Chapter 13. As such, the lymphatic system benefits from general treatment. However, working the specific reflexes of the lymph nodes helps lymph drainage and is useful to include at the end of the treatment.

- OEDEMA – swelling caused by excess fluid from the circulatory system which has accumulated within the tissue. *Direct reflex* = affected area and corresponding lymph node. *Indirect reflexes* = other lymph nodes.

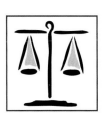

Remember

The working of specific body systems may be applied in any order.

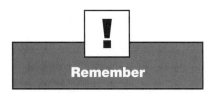

Tip

To test that an oedema is related to fluid retention, press a finger upon the affected area. The surface should pit and slowly regain its original contour.

Holistic harmony

The lymphatic system provides a pick up and cleaning service for the body by collecting fluid and removing waste and harmful substances. By doing this it forms a vital part of the immune system of the body, assisting in its defence mechanisms. As with all of the systems of the body, the lymphatic system relies on the harmony between systems for its well-being and an integration of functions for the well-being of the body as a whole.

Air

Breathing helps the general flow of lymph through the vessels. The bellowing action of the lungs helps to massage the thoracic duct stimulating lymphatic drainage. Deep breathing causes a variation of pressure in the lungs which adds to the stimulating effect. Lymphatic flow is speeded up and the removal of waste is more efficient. This action assists in the prevention of a build up of waste in the body helping to avoid localised **oedema** (swelling). Incorporating deep breathing at the start of the reflexology treatment provides an effective means to improve lymphatic flow, whilst deep breathing at the close of the treatment helps lymphatic drainage.

Water

The volume of lymph in the body is affected by the amount of fluid taken in. Dehydration results in static lymph which disturbs and hinders the normal flow resulting in localised puffiness and oedema (swelling). Water is the solvent of the body responsible for regulating the activity of the solutes it dissolves and circulates and is therefore vital if this function is to be effective and efficient.

Lack of water is a contributory factor in the development of cellulite. Lymphatic circulation becomes sluggish and lymphatic vessels become congested, resulting in the appearance of dimpled skin that takes on an orange peel effect. Cellulite tends to occur in the legs of women, where sluggish lymphatic circulation is common, and may be linked to the effects of the menstrual cycle.

Nutrition

The lymphatic system is instrumental in maintaining the body's immunity through its defending functions. Immunity is maintained by a balanced intake of nutrients including:

- Protein for the production of macrophage cells and lymphocytes for the filtering and destruction of antigens.
- Unsaturated fats in favour of saturated fats that clog up lymphatic vessels.
- Antioxidants – vitamins A, C, and E for their protection against free radicals.
- Minerals such as zinc for its immune-boosting properties and selenium for its immune-enhancing effects.

Additional natural immune-boosting supplements that are in popular use include:

- Aloe vera – antiviral and antiseptic.
- Echinacea – antiviral and anti-bacterial.

Fascinating Fact

A 20-minute afternoon nap can dramatically improve the way the body functions. Any longer sends a person into a deep sleep that will leave them feeling groggy when they awake.

Rest

Lymph flow has to defy gravity on its route back up the body from the arms and legs to the nodes and ducts. In order to rest, the postural muscles relax and the body feels the need to lie down. This brings about an even physical state whereby the flow of lymph is aided. In addition, rest also aids venous blood flow which works in the same way as lymphatic flow. Regular periods of rest ensure a more efficient free flow of lymph and venous blood helping to avoid oedema (swelling) and the associated pain.

Activity

Lymphatic circulation together with venous blood circulation relies heavily on the physical activity of the body. Unlike arterial blood, venous blood and lymph circulate through the body without the aid of the heart acting as a pump. Veins and lymphatic vessels rely on the action of the skeletal muscles to force their contents through the systems. A certain amount of regular exercise is therefore of prime importance for the regulation of circulation to avoid a build up of static lymph. In addition, regular exercise contributes to the avoidance of cellulite.

Circulation of venous blood and lymph in the legs is further hindered by excessive weight. This puts additional pressure on the circulation making it difficult for free flow and as a result, swelling in the legs and ankles is common place in overweight people.

Massage can provide an aid to the circulation of lymph, with movements being directed with pressure in the direction of flow towards lymph nodes and ducts which in turn helps direct venous blood flow back to the heart.

Tip

Lying down with the legs raised helps lymphatic flow as the natural pull of gravity is reversed.

Age

As the body slows down with age so does lymphatic circulation and function. Care should therefore be taken to pay special attention to all of the factors that stimulate circulation and boost the functions of the lymphatic system. Reflexology can further enhance these activities, by helping to balance the system and in turn the rest of the body. Remembering that each body system is in some way reliant on the other systems for its well-being can be the key to anti-ageing. Caring for the whole body is a much more efficient way of caring for the part rather than localised, isolated care that does not integrate the systems.

Awareness

The lymphatic system provides an additional route for the return of interstitial fluid to the blood and lymphatic vessels are present in all tissues and organs of the body except for:

- The central nervous system
- The cornea of the eye
- The internal ear
- The epidermis of the skin
- Cartilage
- Bone marrow.

These areas rely solely on venous blood flow to remove excess fluid and waste.

The lymphatic system acts as a passive drainage system, eventually returning the interstitial fluid to the bloodstream.

Lymph nodes are situated at strategic points along the route formed by the lymphatic vessels and provide a sampling of the fluid lymph for bacteria, viruses and foreign particles. Specific nodes filter lymph from certain areas of the body and include:

- Cervical nodes situated in the neck filter lymph from the head and neck.
- Axillary nodes situated in the armpit filter lymph from the upper arms and upper areas of the trunk.
- Inguinal nodes situated in the groin filter lymph from the lower limbs.

In addition, the areas of lymphatic tissue provide a general filtration effect with:

- The spleen filtering blood.
- The adenoids and tonsils in the pharynx filtering incoming air, water and food.
- The appendix and Peyer's patches filtering waste in the intestines.

An awareness of the position and function of these structures helps in the understanding of the problems that can occur within the lymphatic system as well as create a greater appreciation of the possible causes of malfunction.

Special care

The lymphatic system provides a set of channels for the collection of waste along with venous blood circulation for elimination out of the body.

The elimination systems of the body include:

- The respiratory system for the elimination of waste products associated with respiration e.g. carbon dioxide.
- The digestive system for the elimination of the waste products associated with digestion i.e. faeces.
- The urinary system for the elimination of the waste products associated with cellular function e.g. the formation of urine in the kidneys as a result of filtration of the blood.
- The skin for the elimination of waste products through sweating.

In the same way as the body benefits from what is put into it by means of air, water and food, there is also great value in its output functions in terms of breathing, defecating, urinating and sweating. A balance in output and input is the key to health and well-being and special care should be given to all of these functions.

Remember

The waste products filtered from lymph in the nodes and tissues will be taken to the kidneys by the blood for excretion in urine.

Angel advice

The body automatically adjusts the elimination functions associated with breathing and sweating, however it alerts us to the need to eliminate faeces and urine and relies on our cooperation! Lack of cooperation leads to localised stress as the organs of the digestive and urinary system suffer, as well as general stress through the knock-on effect of linked systems.

Case study

Aspects of the lymphatic system are a part of every other system of the body and one question that is always asked is whether or not a particular organ or gland that has been removed from the body can be detected through reflexology. The medical profession believe that the human body can adapt to the removal of certain organs and glands and it will often emerge during the consultation that a client has had perhaps their appendix, tonsils or adenoids removed. In addition, it is also fairly common for clients to have had other organ/glands removed e.g. gall bladder, ovaries etc.

It is useful to consider the effects on the body of the removal of a particular organ or gland, in terms of the loss of its function and the possible trauma to the surrounding area as a result of the removal procedure. As a result, it may be that a difference in texture and tone may be felt by the practitioner when working over the corresponding area on the feet/hands/ears. It would be unreasonable to expect to pick up on the fact that removal of the organ/gland had taken place without prior knowledge from the client. Sometimes a client will forget certain things during the consultation and it may be that the practitioner is alerted to a reflex point but cannot understand why. Careful questioning of the client often reveals a previous operation many years ago from which they suffer no adverse effects and so tend to forget it ever happened until reminded. In this case the reflexology treatment has alerted the practitioner to the specific area of the body but it cannot always be expected to know the reasons why. Clients often come for a treatment with the misconception that reflexology can diagnose and cure. It is important to ensure that each client is aware of the limits of the treatment and that a realistic set of objectives is agreed at the onset.

Task

Using the treatment card as a guide work the reflexes for the lymphatic system on the feet, hands or ears noting the areas and levels of stress. Begin with a consultation (new or updated), continue with relaxation movements and incorporate the treatment of the previous systems for practice. Finish with relaxation movements, breathing exercises, feedback and aftercare advice.

Knowledge review

1   What is lymph?

2   Name the lymph nodes located in the underarm, groin and neck.

3   Where is the spleen located in the body and what is it responsible for?

4   What does the thymus gland produce and why?

5   Name the two lymphatic ducts.

6   What do the lymphatic ducts drain into?

7   What are the three functions of the lymphatic system?

8   Where is the reflex area for the breast on the feet?

9   Where is the reflex point for the inguinal lymph nodes located on the hands?

10   What are the benefits of drainage movements of the ear reflex points for the spine and joints?

Conclusion

Angel advice

Well done: you now know the whole routine! Continue to practise using the treatment card as a guide, changing the order of work as required.

The journey from having an initial interest in reflexology to being a competent practitioner is one of physical, mental and often spiritual challenges.

The information in this book is designed to encourage an open-minded outlook to the possibilities of reflexology – appreciate and question the many treatment variations whilst at the same time learning to justify your own beliefs.

Learning is not completed on reading the last page of one book or indeed on gaining a qualification, and although the path followed through a book and the study of a course is often long and hard it does not signify the end but rather the beginning. I hope that you enjoy the rest of your journey and that this book continues to be a source of learning and inspiration as you follow your own path.

Glossary

acute used to describe a condition that is sudden, severe and short in duration

adenoids lymphatic tissue in the throat

adrenal glands endocrine glands situated above the kidneys

adrenalin hormone produced by the adrenal glands in response to stress

affirmation positive words to 'voice' intent

aldosterone hormone produced in the adrenal glands controlling the levels of salts in the blood

alveoli tiny air sacs in the lungs where the interchange of gases takes place

anatomy structure

androgens male hormones

andropause male menopause

anterior front

antidiuretic hormone hormone produced in the pituitary gland to control water levels in the body

antioxidants nutrients that counteract free radical attack e.g. vitamins A, C and E

antigen harmful substance

anus final part of the large intestine

apical breathing shallow breathing

appendix lymphatic tissue in the digestive system

arteries blood vessels leading away from the heart

auditory canal internal portion of the ear

auditory types associated with right brain activity

aura human energy field

aural by ear

auricle earflap or pinna

autonomic nervous system sympathetic and parasympathetic nervous systems responsible for automatic functions

axon nerve fibres which carry impulses away from the cell body

balancing to bring about a state of equilibrium

bile secretion of the liver which is stored in the gall bladder

blood pressure pumping action of the heart

bone marrow red bone marrow is found in cancellous bone and is responsible for the formation of new blood cells. Yellow bone marrow is made up of fat cells and is stored in the length of some compact bone

bronchi air passageways leading into the lungs

bronchioles small air passageways in the lungs

caecum start of the large intestine

calcitonin hormone produced in the thyroid gland

cancellous bone spongy bone tissue

capillaries single cell structures at the end of blood and lymph vessels

carbohydrates energy-producing foods

carbon dioxide gas produced in the cells as a result of using oxygen

cardiac muscular tissue muscle tissue exclusive to the heart

cardiac sphincter ring of muscle between the oesophagus and the stomach

carpals bones of the wrist

cartilage connective tissue providing additional support for the skeletal system

cartilaginous joints slightly moveable joints

case history details gained during a consultation relating to personal, medical, physical, emotional and lifestyle factors

catabolism chemical reaction within a cell that causes the break down of nutrients into the smallest possible form for energy production

cell microscopic part of an organ

central nervous system the brain and spinal cord

cerebral hemispheres left and right halves of the brain

cerebrum the forebrain

cerumen earwax

cervical vertebrae the seven bones of the spine forming the neck

chakras energy centres

chi traditional Chinese term for energy

chronic term used to describe a condition which is long in duration

chyme broken-down food in the stomach

cilia tiny hairs attached to a cell

circulatory systems transport systems for blood and lymph

clavicle collar bone

coccyx the four fused bones of the spine forming the tail bone

code of ethics a specific set of rules laid down by a regulatory body

collagen protein found in connective tissue e.g. skin, bones

colon large intestine

communication a means to convey a message

compact bone hard bone tissue

conception vessel controlling vessel of yin meridians

connective tissue groups of cells forming a protective and supportive tissue

consultation establishing whether or not a client is suitable for treatment. A consultation forms a continuous and progressive part of the reflexology treatment

contra action an adverse reaction to a treatment, a disturbance of state

contraindication a condition which could be made worse by treatment or be a possible cause of cross infection

cortisol mineralocorticoid produced in the adrenal glands

COSHH Control of Substances Hazardous to Health Regulations 1999

counselling a way of conveying a message in a helpful manner

cranial nerves twelve pairs of nerves coming from the brain to all parts of the face

cranium the head

cupping a form of percussion massage

dehydration lack of moisture

dendrite nerve fibre which passes impulses to the cell body

deoxygenated lacking in oxygen

dermatoglyphics the study of the patterns of the skin of the palms of the hands and fingers and the soles of the feet and toes

dermatomes segmented regions of the body each of which are supplied with a nerve

dermis layer of connective tissue below the epidermis of the skin

diaphragm muscle separating the abdomen and the thorax

diaphragmatic breathing deep breathing

digestive system responsible for the intake of nutrients and the release of waste

distal the point furthest away from an attachment

diuretic a substance that increases urine production

dorsal back or posterior surface

ducts tubes

duodenum first part of the small intestine

effleurage smoothing, surface massage movements

empathy understanding another person's feelings

endocrine system responsible for controlling the body through chemical messengers in the form of hormones secreted by endocrine glands

epidermis top layer of skin

epithelial tissue groups of cells forming layers of protective tissue

eustachian tube connecting the middle ear with the nasopharynx

excretion the process of eliminating waste from the body

exhalation breathing out

external auditory meatus auditory canal

faeces waste product of the digestive system

fats foods that provide the body with a source of energy

fertilisation the impregnation of an ovum by a sperm

fibre food which is indigestible and is needed to aid elimination of waste from the digestive system

fibrous joints fixed joints

foetus developing baby

follicle stimulating hormone hormone produced in the pituitary gland which has an effect on the gonads

free radicals the toxic by-product of energy metabolism

frictions a form of petrissage massage

gall bladder accessory organ of the digestive system. Stores bile to aid digestion

genitalia reproductive organs

genito-urinary system the male and female genitalia responsible for reproduction and the urinary organs responsible for helping to maintain the body's fluid balance

gland a structure lined with epithelial tissue which secretes a substance

glucagon hormone produced in the pancreas helping to control blood sugar levels

glycogen the form in which carbohydrates are stored in the muscles and the liver

gonads reproductive organs

governing vessel controlling vessel of yang meridians

growth hormone hormone produced in the pituitary gland

hacking a form of percussion massage

haemoglobin substance that allows the blood cells to carry oxygen and carbon dioxide

HASAWA Health and Safety at Work Act 1974

healing to make or become well

healing crisis extreme reaction, a turning point or danger point characterised by the body's need to get worse before getting better

helix upper section of the ear flap

hepatic flexure bend in the large intestine

holding a method of greeting the feet, hands or ears at the start and finish of a reflexology treatment

holistic considering the complete person, the whole self – body, mind and spirit

homeostasis physiological stability

hook-in-back-up a pressure technique

hormones chemical messengers produced by endocrine glands

human energy field (HEF) energy surrounding living things

hyper secretion oversecretion

hypodermis layer of fatty tissue lying directly below the dermis of the skin

hyposecretion undersecretion

ileocaecal sphincter ring of muscle at the end of the ileum

ileum final part of the large intestine

immune system responsible for protecting the body against disease

infectious a condition that can be passed from person to person

inflammation a localised protective response

inhalation breath in

insulin hormone produced in the pancreas helping to regulate blood sugar levels

integumentary system consisting of the skin, hair and nails

Islets of Langerhans endocrine section of the pancreas

jargon technical terms relating to treatment. Questions directed at the client should be jargon-free

jejunum middle section of the small intestine

joint the point at which two or more bones meet

joint manipulation a type of massage used during relaxation

ki traditional Japanese term for energy

kidneys two bean shaped organs that produce urine

kneading a form of petrissage massage

knuckling a form of petrissage massage

lacteals lymphatic capillaries in the small intestine

larynx upper throat

lateral away from the midline

lateral costal breathing normal breathing

lateral longitudinal arch arch running along the outside edges of the feet

left brain left cerebral hemisphere of the brain associated with analytical functions and logical thinking. Controls the right side of the body

legislative requirements a general set of rules laid down by a government department

leucocytes white blood cells

lifestyle details relating to work, leisure, diet and exercise. Information gained during a consultation

ligaments attach bone to bone at a joint

liver largest organ of the body

longitudinal lengthways

lumbar vertebrae the five bones of the spine forming the lower back

lungs organs of respiration

luteinising hormone hormone produced in the pituitary gland affecting the gonads

lymph straw-coloured fluid

lymphatic tissue connective tissue which forms lymph nodes

lymphocytes white blood cells that produce an antibody against an antigen

macrocosm large system e.g. the human body

mantras special phrases to focus on energy flow within the body

master gland pituitary gland

medial towards the midline

medial longitudinal arch arch running along the inside edges of the feet

meiosis a process of cell reproduction to create a new organism

melanin the natural colour pigment

melanocyte stimulating hormone hormone produced by the pituitary gland affecting the production of melanin in the skin

menopause the cessation of the female menstrual cycle

menstruation the release of an unfertilised ovum from the uterus

meridians energy channels

metabolism a chemical process within the cells

metacarpals bones of the hand

metatarsals bones of the feet

microcosm miniature representation of a larger system

midline the centre line of the body

mineralocorticoids hormones produced in the adrenal glands

minerals food that provides the body with the nutrients needed to perform its functions

mitosis simple cell division

motor nerves receive messages from the central nervous system

mucus fluid formed by goblet cells

muscular system muscles of the body responsible for voluntary and involuntary movement

nadis energy lines in Indian Ayurvedic medicine

nervous system central, peripheral and autonomic nervous systems responsible for controlling the body with electrical impulses

neuron nerve cell

non-verbal communication the use of the body to convey a message

noradrenalin hormone/neurotransmitter produced in the adrenal glands in response to stress

oedema swelling caused by excess fluid in the tissues

oestrogen female hormone produced in the ovaries

olfactory sense of smell

open questions questions that require more than a one word answer

oral spoken

organ a structure that is made up of two or more tissue types and has specific form and function

organism the sum of cells, tissues, organs and body systems

ova eggs

ovum single egg

oxygen vital gas breathed into the body from the air

oxygenated rich in oxygen

oxytocin hormone produced in the pituitary gland affecting the reproductive organs

palpation the examination of a part by touch or pressure of the hand

pancreas accessory organ of digestion. Also has endocrine functions

parathormone hormone produced in the parathyroid glands affecting mineral levels in the blood

parathyroid glands endocrine glands located in the neck along with the thyroid glands

perceptive obtain knowledge through use of the senses

percussion a brisk, stimulating form of massage

periosteum connective tissue forming a protective outer covering to the length of bones

peripheral nervous system 12 pairs of cranial nerves and 31 pairs of spinal nerves

peristalsis involuntary muscular action

petrissage deep massage movements

Peyer's patches lymphatic tissue in the small intestine

phalanges bones of the fingers and toes

pharynx back of the throat

pineal gland endocrine gland situated in the brain

pinna ear flap or auricle

pituitary gland endocrine gland situated in the brain

pivot-on-a-point a pressure technique

plasma fluid part of blood

plexus network of nerves

pounding a form of percussion massage

practitioner a person who performs a skill

prana traditional Indian term for energy

progesterone female hormone produced in the ovaries

prolactin hormone produced in the pituitary gland affecting the gonads

prostate gland produces the fluid part of semen in males as part of the genito-urinary system

proteins food that provides the body with the nutrients for growth and repair

proximal closest point of an attachment

PRS Performing Rights Society

puberty the time when secondary sexual development starts to take place

pulse contraction and relaxation of the heart

pyloric sphincter ring of muscle between the stomach and the duodenum

rectum latter part of the large intestine

reflexes points on the feet, hands and/or ears that reflect organs of the body

respiratory system system responsible for breathing involving the intake of oxygen and release of carbon dioxide

RIDDOR Reporting of Injuries, Diseases and Dangerous Occurrences Regulations 1995

right brain right cerebral hemisphere of the brain associated with systemic functions and creative thinking. Controls the left side of the body

rotation a form of joint manipulation

RSI repetitive strain injury

safe stress high demands, low constraints with high levels of support

secretion a cellular process for releasing a substance

semen secretion from the testes, seminal vesicles and prostate gland containing sperm

seminal vesicles small sac-like structures responsible for secreting the fluid part of semen

sensory nerves carry impulses from the sensory organs to the central nervous system

sex corticoids hormones produced in the adrenal glands

shaking a form of vibration massage

sinuses air spaces in the facial bones containing mucous lining

skeletal muscles voluntary muscles

skeletal system bones and joints of the body

skull bones of the cranium and face

solar plexus network of nerves situated in the abdomen below the diaphragm

spleen lymphatic tissue situated in the upper left side of the abdomen

splenic flexure bend in the large intestine

stress high demands, high constraints with low levels of support

synovial joints freely moveable joints

systemic affecting the body as a whole

tactile sense of touch

tapotement a stimulating form of massage movement

tarsal bones bones of the ankle

tendons attach muscle to bone

testosterone male hormone produced in the testes

thymosins hormones produced by the thymus gland

thymus gland endocrine gland situated behind the sternum

thyroid gland endocrine gland situated in the neck

thyroid stimulating hormone hormone produced in the pituitary galnd affecting the thyroid gland

thyroxine hormone produced in the thyroid gland helping to regulate metabolism

tonsils lymphoid tissue situated in the throat

transverse running across

transverse arch arch running across the balls of the feet

tsubo Japanese meridian points.

tympanic cavity middle ear

tympanic membrane eardrum

universal energy field (UEF) energy living within the world around us

ureters tubes leading from the kidneys to the bladder

urethra tube leading out of the body from the bladder

urinary system responsible for the removal of waste from the body in the formulation of urine

urine water and waste produced in the kidneys

uterus womb

verbal communication the use of the voice to convey a message

vertebrae bones of the spine

vibration a form of massage used during relaxation

visceral muscles involuntary muscles

visual types associated with left brain activity

visualisation the use of positive images and/or colour to bring about physiological changes in the body

vitamins food that provides the body with nutrients to maintain its vital functions

yang energy representing positive active polarity

yin energy representing negative inactive polarity

zones longitudinal or transverse sections through which energy flows

Index

Guildford College
Learning Resource Centre

Please return on or before the last date shown.
No further issues or renewals if any items are overdue.
"7 Day" loans are **NOT** renewable.

2 9 JUN 2004   1 6 OCT 2008

-5 OCT 2004

- 1 NOV 2004

0 4 NOV 2005

1 5 MAR 2006

1 3 DEC 2007

2 5 APR 2008

Class: 615.822 PAR

Title: Holistic Guide to Reflexology

Author: PARSONS, Tina